YOU AND YOUR HORMONES

INTERNATIONAL EDITION

Dr Peter Baratosy MBBS, FACNEM

Dr Peter Baratosy is a registered Medical Doctor in Australia. He graduated from the University of Adelaide Medical School in 1978. He is a Fellow of the Australasian College of Nutritional and Environmental Medicine and is an accredited Medical Acupuncturist with the Medical Board of Australia.

Published by Dr Peter Baratosy 2025

Copyright Dr Peter Baratosy 2025

Original Cover Design Karen English

Modified by Nikola Boskovski

Edited Karen Mace

Formatting Nikola Boskovski

ISBN - 978-0-6451053-9-1 (Print edition)

978-1-7637752-0-6 (e Book)

Dr Peter Baratosy MBBS FACNEM

Dedicated to my darling Jenny. Thank you for all your love, support and encouragement. I could not have achieved this without you.

I also dedicate this book to all those giants on whose shoulders I have stood on. To all the men and women who have done the research and without whom this book could not have been written.

I also dedicate this book to my ACNEM colleagues, from whom I have learned so much.

Finally, this book is dedicated to Mr. and Mrs. B. You know who you are. You told me to write this book on hormones!

Table of Contents

PRE-MENSTRUAL TENSION, PERI-

Part 1

INTRODUCTION

"All truth passes through three stages. First, it is ridiculed. Second, it is violently opposed. Third, it is accepted as being self-evident."

Arthur Schopenhauer (1788-1860)
German Philosopher

"Modern medicine is not scientific. It is full of prejudice, illogic and susceptible to advertising. Doctors are not taught to reason; they are programmed to believe in whatever their medical schools teach them, and the leading doctors tell them. Over the past 20 years, the drug companies, with their enormous wealth, have taken medicine over and now control its research, what is taught and the information released to the public."

Abram Hoffer (1917–2009)
Canadian biochemist, physician and psychiatrist

For many years, mainstream doctors have ridiculed, teased, derided, criticized, and mocked practitioners who used transdermal natural hormones instead of the pharmaceutical oral synthetic hormones. All sorts of excuses were thrown about.

- They are dangerous.
- They do not work.
- Transdermal creams do not absorb adequately.

However, newer studies show that these natural hormones are safer, and the transdermal creams do absorb adequately. The synthetic hormones are more dangerous.

The ironic thing is that the mainstream is now using more natural hormones and nearly all hormones are being given transdermally as gels, creams, or patches! (See Schopenhauer)

In this book, I will discuss research on hormones, specifically the synthetic hormones (hormone replacement therapy - HRT) and why the natural bio-identical hormone replacement therapy (B-HRT) is safer and therefore more appropriate.

Another reason for this book is to show that there are other ways of treating hormonal problems in men and women, other than just supplementing hormones.

We can replace hormones, but one question we should ask is, *"Why do hormones decline or become imbalanced in the first place?"*

The ageing process, of course, is one reason: but there is also the pollution, the poor western diet, the stresses, in fact, nearly all aspects of western civilized living can affect our health which, in turn, can affect our hormones, or *vice versa*.

If we use the diet, nutrition, herbs, etc. we may make a difference. If hormones need to be replaced, then bio-identical hormone replacement should be the preference for safety reasons.

Before I start, perhaps it would be a good idea to define the terminology I use in what I will be discussing. This is important because the basis of much of the confusion is a matter of semantics; that is nomenclature.

The word *natural* has been used in many ways. However, in this book, when I use the word *"natural"*, it means I am referring to the molecule that is exactly the same as the one made by the body.

Another word that I use frequently is "bio-identical", meaning "biologically identical". The word "bio-identical" has been derided by the mainstream as just a "marketing tool" to make people think that there is something special about what is being promoted. In fact, there *is* something special about such a hormone, it is the same as that which is made by Mother Nature: so, it must be special! Mother Nature would not have designed a specific molecule unless it was the most appropriate for the job.

In this book, I will use the terms *bio-identical* and *natural* interchangeably, both describing hormones which have the same structure as those made by the body.

Drug companies are producing a similar molecule and promoting their synthetic, new to nature drug to be the best and preferable to what is natural.

Not only do they have the audacity to say that these synthetic similar molecules are better and safer than the natural molecule, they also then go one step further and try to convince the population that the natural molecules are dangerous.

Natural molecules are only dangerous to their profits.

> Bio-identical = natural = the same molecule as that which is made by the body.

Drug company hormones differ from natural hormones. The natural oestrogen made by the body is 17-beta-oestradiol. The oestrogens produced by drug companies are *not* 17-beta-oestradiol: they are ethinyl-estradiol, mestranol, dienestrol, quinestrol, polyestradiol phosphate, diethylstilbestrol (DES), estropipate and many more; these are definitely *not* 17-beta-oestradiol.

The word "bio-identical" is not a marketing tool, it is a *descriptive* term. A term used to describe that the molecule is the same molecule as that which is made by the body.

The body naturally makes various hormones that are molecularly unique, and it makes sense that these same molecules, instead of something similar, should be used when replacing hormones.

When I use the word *"synthetic"* I am referring to hormones manufactured by the drug companies that are *not* the same as the natural hormones; they have been altered in some way. They are similar, but not exact.

The term "synthesised" can also be confusing. Synthesised is just another word meaning "made" or "manufactured". Even the natural, bio-identical hormones are "synthesised", that is, they are manufactured. The starting point is usually a molecule (e.g. diosgenin) from a plant such as Mexican wild yam

(*Dioscorea villosa*), which is then further converted in a laboratory. The critical issue here is the structure of the end product; it doesn't matter how it is made, but the end result should be a molecule that is exactly the same as that made by the body.

There are many hormones naturally produced in the body, such as oestrogen, progesterone, testosterone, melatonin, cortisol, dehydroepiandrosterone (DHEA) and thyroid hormone. All these have a specific structure.

The drug companies have altered some of these hormones, which means that they can now be patented for commercial purposes. As we shall see, these synthetic analogues have a long list of side effects that generally do not occur with the original natural hormones. If side effects do develop with the natural hormones, it is to a far lesser extent, and possibly because of poor prescribing.

Since the use of these natural hormones is not taught in medical schools, only those enlightened doctors who have studied a more natural form of medicine are aware of them. These hormones can only be made up and dispensed by compounding pharmacists.

"Compounding is the process of making a medication from raw ingredients that are either not readily available on the Australian market, currently

out of stock or were not manufactured in the precise dose and/or dosage form that you have been prescribed."

(https://www.freshtherapeutics.com.au › what-is-a-compounding-pharmacy Accessed 20 May 2024)

Compounding pharmacists make products in different forms such as creams, troche, suppository, or pessary. They also make up natural hormones as prescribed by the doctor.

We have the "natural" hormones, and we have the "synthetic" hormones. Since we are classifying hormones, we can mention a third category, a category where the hormones are "natural" but are from a different species.

While they are "natural" for that species, they are totally inappropriate for use in humans. Here I am referring specifically to *conjugated equine estrogen* (CEE). This is a hormone product made from pregnant horse's urine.

What were they thinking when they decided to use horse's urine? Though note that pregnant mare's urine does contain significant levels of oestrogen.

What is even more troubling is that the women using this product and possibly even the doctors prescribing it did not know its source.

An interesting question *"What if these women were vegans or vegetarians?"* Would that have been an issue?

Wherever possible, if hormones are needed and used, the natural, bio-identical should be used.

SEX HORMONES

Oestrogen

A woman has three main oestrogens,

1) oestradiol (10-20%),
2) oestriol (60-80%), and
3) oestrone (10-20%).

Women need these specific hormones and not something similar. They definitely do not need horse hormones!

In the past, one of the most popular forms of hormone replacement therapy (HRT) used conjugated equine estrogen (CEE), which was derived from horse urine. CEE contains oestrone (75-80%), equilin (6-15%), as well as oestradiol plus others (5-19%). This product is still available, though thankfully is not being prescribed as much.

The drug company making this product is using the word "natural" in describing the product. I do not want to mention specific drug companies or products. However, this product, promoted as natural in a way that could be construed as misleading to believe it is natural in the human context, comes from **pregnant mare's urine**.

Yes, it is a natural product. It is a biological identical hormone … for horses!

While this product has some similarities to human hormones, it is still an inappropriate product for humans. As we shall see, similarity is not good enough.

Equilin is a true horse oestrogen and has a much more potent oestrogenic action than human oestrogen. As noted above, CEE contains the wrong oestrogens, the wrong potencies and, in the wrong proportions. Why then should women have to use such a product?

Hormones and their receptors are like a key and a lock. Even the slightest change can make a huge difference. Imagine a set of keys; while they all look very similar, if you try to open a lock with the wrong key, it won't work. However, if you do manage to open the lock - with some force - damage probably will occur.

So, it is with oestrogens: synthetic or from another species. They may be similar; they may seem to work superficially but they have many side effects. This is what we see in clinical practice.

Diethylstilbesterol (DES)

Although diethylstilbesterol (DES) does not possess a steroidal structure like an oestrogen, it has extremely strong oestrogenic properties. This compound was used extensively between 1938 and the 1970s to "prevent miscarriage". Not only was it found to be useless, but the women taking the drug developed significant side effects such as thromboses, fluid retention, breast tenderness, loss of libido, tiredness, nausea, weight gain, headaches and hair thinning. These women also developed an increased incidence of breast cancer, though not of other hormone sensitive tissues, such as endometrium or ovary (Titus-Ernstoff et al., 2001).

Many thousands of unborn children were exposed to this drug. The daughters developed cancer later, specifically clear cell adenocarcinoma of the vagina, while the boys developed congenital reproductive tract abnormalities, notably hypospadias (Klip et al., 2002).

The daughters of DES women also have a high incidence of reproductive dysfunction (Titus-Ernstoff et al., 2006), as well as an increased risk of breast cancer, specifically in the over 40 age group (Palmer et al., 2006).

It is evident from these studies that the side effects may only become apparent after a long period of time.

There is also some evidence that the generation after, the third generation, can also be affected (Blatt, Van Le, Weiner & Sailer, 2003).

This raises the question of trans-generational DES-related epigenetic alterations in humans (Titus-Ernstoff et al. 2006).

Examples of synthetic oestrogens

- ethinyl-estradiol,
- diethylstilbestrol (DES),
- estropipate, mestranol,
- dienestrol,
- quinestrol,
- polyestradiol phosphate,
- conjugated equine estrogen (CEE)–estrogen made from horse urine.

Progesterone

Progesterone is one specific molecule.

If the structure is changed, even slightly, then it is *not* progesterone; it may have progestogenic activity, but it is *not* progesterone. This is what we refer to as a *progestin*.

Nomenclature: this would be an opportune time to define a few terms that will appear from time to time in this book.

A *progestogen* or *progestin* is a molecule that has progestogenic activity. The natural progestogen made by the human body is *progesterone*.

An example of a progestin is medroxyprogesterone acetate (MPA).

This point must be emphasised because during researching this book, I have seen many times where *"progesterone"* is interchanged with *"progestin"*.

I have spoken with drug representatives (drug reps) who tell me that their product contains progesterone. When I confront them, some sheepishly admit that it is not progesterone but a progestin. Others

25

did not seem to know the difference, or really care.

Even some researchers do not seem to know the difference, as some published papers mix up progesterone with progestins.

Confusing?

Yes!

Irritating?

Definitely!

Examples of progestins

- norethisterone,
- norethynodrel,
- norethindrone,
- norgestimate,
- norgestrel,
- levonorgestrel,
- medroxyprogesterone,
- desogestrel,
- drospirenone

Testosterone

Testosterone, again, is one specific molecule and, like the others discussed above, has also been altered and patented.

Men need testosterone, and it may seem hard to believe, but women also need some testosterone, which is often thought of as the "male hormone". Women make and need about one tenth the amount of men. One tenth does seem like a small amount, but that small amount *is* needed.

Women with various issues, such as heart disease, bladder incontinence and osteoporosis, can be treated with physiological doses of testosterone.

Testosterone in women has also been shown to improve libido, motivation, and mood.

Examples of synthetic testosterone

- fluoxymesterone,
- nandrolone,
- danozol,
- oxymetholone,
- oxandrolone.

Testosterone can also be esterified, allowing a long-lasting effect on injection, e.g. testosterone cypionate. Testosterone can also be alkalinised, substituting a methyl group or an ethyl group for the hydroxyl group. This allows for oral dosing. An example is methyltestosterone.

Both men and women need testosterone, although in different doses. Preferably, the natural, bio-identical form, in a physiological dose, should be used; not something synthetic and similar.

SYNTHETIC HORMONES

Hormone structures and shapes are very specific: any minor change can produce vastly different effects.

This is exemplified by the fact that the difference between oestrogen and testosterone, between male and female, is only one hydrogen atom and a double bond.

That little variation does make such a big difference!

"Vive la différence."

Drug companies make hormones that are not the identical, original type. Due to legislation, natural molecules *cannot* be patented. This means that any natural molecule needs to be modified so that the giant multi-national drug company can profit from it. Of course, even if any big drug company did spend millions of dollars on doing the research on a natural molecule, in the end, they would not be able to patent the product. Other companies could use that research and manufacture that same product, because the molecule, being natural, *cannot* be patented.

No company should ever hold a patent on a molecule made by nature.

This is probably the main reason there is little incentive to research natural products.

This inability to patent natural molecules is one of the main reasons why drug companies make alterations to a natural molecule. By inventing a molecule *like* the natural molecule, similar - but unique enough to be different and therefore not natural, they can then patent this new similar molecule and exploit it. The drug companies use an expensive advertising campaign purchased by their wealth and power to encourage the population to use their newly patented, similar, and expensive hormone products.

The manufactured molecule is similar, but not exactly the same as the natural molecule. Since these new, invented molecules are new to nature, long-term, double-blind studies *must* be done because they are new to nature. No one knows, nor can predict, what effect they have on human physiology. With hormones, even the smallest changes do make big differences: remember that the difference between oestrogen and testosterone, the difference between man and woman, is only one hydrogen atom and a double bond. Therefore, there must be a lot of research on these synthetic altered molecules to see what effects such molecules have on the human physiology.

We can argue that long-term double-blind studies do not need to be done on natural molecules because we already know their action, we can predict what they do. Studies on natural molecules are studies on *normal physiology* and have been carried out for many years. The results are what we read in physiology textbooks.

As I have already stated, hormones and their receptors are like a lock and a key. The natural key fits perfectly into the lock and the lock opens. However, if you use a similar key, you may, with a bit of forcing, open the lock, but there is likely to be damage. Conversely, a similar hormone may act as a natural hormone blocker by occupying the receptor and preventing the natural hormone from having its action.

A synthetic similar hormone does a similar job and has a long list of side effects.

Unfortunately, the natural hormones and the synthetic hormones are often lumped together and treated as one. They are not the same and need to be looked at separately.

Now here is the problem.

As mentioned earlier, big pharmaceutical companies want to make money, and they realised that they could make a lot of money by manufacturing a product similar to the natural hormones made by the body.

Now, I'm sure if one of the CEOs or a shareholder of a drug company took their Rolls-Royce, Mercedes, or BMW in for a service and non-genuine replacement parts were used (something similar), I would think that they would get rather upset. So, why should the human body be any different?

There is no need for anyone to use the synthetic (non-identical) analogue hormones (HRT) and not the natural (genuine replacement parts) bio-identical hormones (B-HRT).

In 2002, when the negative results of the Woman's Health Initiative Trial (WHI) were released, thousands of women stopped their synthetic HRT. The results clearly demonstrated that the synthetic hormones were causing more harm than good. Many women taking the products developed conditions such as breast cancer, blood clots in the lung, heart attacks, strokes and dementia. Sales of the most popular synthetic hormone preparations fell by 68%.

Drug companies must have had warehouses full of these products and couldn't even give them away because women just stopped taking them. These women voted with their feet, and many changed to using the natural, bio-identical hormones.

Women's Health Initiative (WHI)

I mentioned the Women's Health Initiative (WHI) above and now is a good time to expand on this study.

The WHI was a study of 161,809 post-menopausal women with intact uteri (Rossouw et al., 2002).

There were many aspects to this study and the relevant part to this section was the combined oestrogen/progestin arm of the trial. The conclusion was that the health risks exceeded benefits from the use of combined oestrogen and progestin over an average of 5.2 years' follow up. There was an increase in breast cancer, heart attacks, strokes, and pulmonary emboli. The study was stopped early because of a statistical increase in breast cancer and stroke and no benefit from reducing cardiovascular risk.

Short-term use was safe for the alleviation of hot flushes, but long-term use caused more morbidity and death than it saved.

Another similar study, the *"Million Women Study"* released soon afterwards, confirmed these findings. Beral et al. (2003) showed that HRT is dangerous for women. At present, the only recommended use for HRT is for short term (under 5 years) treatment of hot flushes (although as we shall see, there are many natural treatments that are a lot safer and can deal with these issues). This study not only showed that oestrogen was dangerous, but the (synthetic) oestrogen and progestin combination was even worse.

Breast cancer rates had been increasing but, in 2003, the rates started to drop in the over 50 age group and have continued to drop. So, what happened in 2003? This is the year that the WHI study was released and made front page in nearly every newspaper in the world. Women were frightened, and rightly so. Up to 46% of women stopped taking the HRT.

Katalinic and Rawal (2008) agree that this reduction of breast cancer rates is most likely because hundreds of thousands of women stopped taking HRT. It is not due to any new treatments.

Ravdin et al. (2007) concurred, *"The decrease was*

evident only in women who were 50 years of age or older and was more evident in cancers that were estrogen–receptor–positive than in those that were estrogen–receptor–negative. The decrease in breast-cancer incidence seems to be temporally related to the first report of the Women's Health Initiative and the ensuing drop in the use of hormone-replacement therapy among postmenopausal women in the United States."

Even the *Adelaide Advertiser* had a say.

"Breast Cancer Rates Decline" says the *Adelaide Advertiser (2 June 2008 pg. 9).*

"Breast cancer rates have fallen because fewer women are using hormone replacement therapy, the latest research shows."

Since synthetic hormones are dangerous, what can we use to treat women? The drug companies want us to think that there are no alternatives. They also want us to think that the natural hormones do not work, or even worse, are dangerous.

Much misinformation about natural hormones has been disseminated, creating panic and confusion. However, most of this misinformation comes from drug companies and their agents, and most is not strictly correct.

How can a natural hormone be dangerous? How is it that a hormone made by our bodies is dangerous? Here, we must differentiate between *physiological* and *pharmacological* uses of hormones.

Take note: I will make the point here and this should be considered throughout the whole book. When I say natural hormones are not, or at least, less dangerous, I am referring specifically to *physiological* replacement. That is, using doses of the natural hormone that will provide physiological levels in the body.

As an extension to this, it also means that the prescriptions are written by doctors who have studied bio-identical hormone replacement therapy (B-HRT). It also means that appropriate doses are prescribed, the levels are monitored, and that the prescription is made up by competent compounding pharmacists.

Any substance can be dangerous in inappropriate doses. Take water, for instance. Too little water and we die of thirst. Too much water, we die from drowning. The same with oxygen. Too much is poisonous, too little is fatal; we need the right amount.

Not too little, not too much! The "Goldilocks' Zone"!

Being told that the natural form of the hormone is dangerous does not make sense. A hormone that is physiological, a natural part of human physiology, is dangerous, yet similar, manufactured (patented and profiting the company) hormones are safe!

How bizarre! This does not make sense.

They make the point that synthetic hormones have been thoroughly researched using various trials and other studies. To a degree, this is correct. The new, altered hormones *had* to be tested to see what they could do.

Drug company sponsored studies are suspect from the start. The funding is from the company therefore, studies are carried out by scientists who cannot be considered unbiased, and it is well known that the drug companies will only release studies that are favourable to their products. As we shall see, some of these studies were written by ghost-writers.

Initially, there were very few trials on natural hormones because no one would fund them, as natural hormones cannot be patented. Fortunately, more studies have now been done.

On the other hand, why do we have to do such studies on natural hormones? Studies on natural hormones have been done for a very long time; it is called physiology. Look up any physiology textbook and you will see the workings and actions of natural

Dr Peter Baratosy MBBS FACNEM

hormones.

Studies have now been done which compare natural hormones with the synthetic hormones. These studies show that natural is always safer than synthetic.

Natural hormones are much safer than synthetic hormones.

I remember quite vividly when the results of the WHI study were released: "HRT CAUSES BREAST CANCER" screamed from nearly every newspaper front page all over the world. The TV and the radio also made comment, and women were scared; and rightly so. Many tossed their HRT into the bin.

I was listening to some of my colleagues discuss the issue in the clinic lunchroom; they were scared just as the drug companies were scared–but for different reasons. The drug companies were worried about dropping profits. My colleagues were worried about their patients.

What were they to do with those patients who were on HRT? How would they now treat their menopausal patients?

I smiled to myself, as I did not have that problem. Most of my patients were either on herbs and nutrients and/or on B-HRT, the real, natural hormones, which did not have these problems. I was aware from the beginning, that the natural hormones had to be much safer by virtue of them being truly natural. Many of my patients thanked me afterwards for knowing about the problem with synthetics and for starting them on the natural hormones.

After the scare, more and more women went on to natural hormones. However, unfortunately, the average conventional doctor does not know anything about natural hormones because,

1) the topic was never taught in Medical School, and
2) the drug reps were continually talking up the synthetic hormones and talking down the natural hormones.

I specifically mention drug reps, because many doctors get a large part of their information/education from these people; I consider them a very biased source, as their job is to promote what the drug company makes.

Women are smart, they think and research, especially about their own health. Many stopped the HRT out of fear, but soon after, when symptoms reappeared, they knew that they couldn't go back on the synthetics. They researched and found out about the natural hormones and actively sought out those few doctors who prescribed them.

Of course, opposition came. Drug companies minimised the results of the WHI and tried to get women back onto synthetic HRT. Misinformation was spread about the dangers and/or ineffectiveness of the "natural" hormones.

Quick history lesson

Why should women need to take hormones, anyway?

Many years ago, in January 1964, a New York gynaecologist, Dr Robert Wilson, wrote an article in Newsweek titled *No More Menopause*. Later, in 1966, he wrote a book called 'Feminine Forever,' which became a best seller. He and his book are reputed to have been sponsored by the drug companies that manufacture synthetic oestrogen products. In the book, he praises the virtues of replacing oestrogen. He likened older women to a *"dried up prune"*; another term he used was that women were in a *"living decay"*, thus needing oestrogen to become young again. His attitude was certainly very misogynistic, and there was a mixed reaction to this from the feminists.

Houck (2003) wrote that *"Between 1963 and 1980, feminists did not respond with one voice to Wilson's ideas: at first, some embraced them as a boon for aging women, while others resisted regarding female aging as pathological."*

He converted menopause, a natural physiological phase of life, into a deficiency disease and perpetuated the myth that menopause is *solely* an oestrogen deficiency disease. He argued that since menopause is a deficiency disease, it could therefore be treated by replacing oestrogen.

Menopause was medicalised.

The book promised women that they could be "feminine forever". This had the connotation of oestrogen being a "youth pill", which certainly hit a chord with many women. Yet the evidence was minimal. This was suggestion and theory, not science. This was a triumph of marketing over science.

Drug companies continued to support him; after all, they could see huge profits.

There is some evidence that it was actually the drug companies that found him and set him up to write the book with studies contracted and paid for by drug companies.

The drug companies were even reputed to have bought large numbers of the book to push it into the "best seller" list.

The Wilson Foundation was set up, again reputedly with funds from drug companies, to promote unopposed oestrogen replacement.

(O) Estrogen Replacement Therapy (ERT) became very popular - no wonder with what it promised! The topic reached the chat shows, the women's magazines, and so on, and many women read his book. Of course, as expected, many of these women went straight to their doctors and demanded to be put on those "wonder pills"; which is what the drug companies hoped for!

Many doctors did.

(O)estrogen Replacement Therapy (ERT) took off with minimal studies but with maximum hype, maximum spin, and maximum PR. It became one of the biggest money spinners for the drug companies.

Too bad the science wasn't there.

Bad news came in 1975 when Smith, Prentice, Thompson, and Herrmann found increased rates of endometrial cancer in women on oestrogen. The rate was seven and a half times greater in ERT users. Women who used ERT for seven years or longer had a 14 times greater chance of developing cancer of the uterus (womb).

Unopposed oestrogen (the use of oestrogen on its own) is possibly the only cause of endometrial cancer. Other side effects included gallbladder disease, fibroids and breast and ovarian cancer.

Women stopped ERT, and sales and profits fell.

The USA Food and Drug Administration (FDA) demanded that all oestrogen products carry an insert warning of its dangers and also demanded that the companies reduced the "youth pill" advertising.

The strange thing was that the American Medical Association (AMA) in conjunction with the drug companies, went to court to resist this demand. They argued that this demand would "unnecessarily frighten women"!

The drug companies did make changes. They made some changes to the product but did not do any new studies. They did, however, hire new PR company and changed their advertising.

They added a substance that could protect the

lining of the uterus. This was a substance that had progestogenic activity. Of course, they did *not* use natural progesterone but added a synthetic, patented progestin and they re-named the product - they now called it hormone replacement therapy (HRT).

A new product, a new name, a new image.

This again required a large amount of spin and hype and PR (although little science) and the profits started to increase again.

The drug companies funded study after study, although possibly only releasing the positive studies. Information about the positive benefits of HRT was channelled to journalists from various "independent foundations" which, in reality, were fronts funded by drug companies.

Colditz et al. (1995) followed up on the "Nurses' Health Study" and showed a greater incidence of breast cancer in the HRT users. The chance of developing breast cancer amongst HRT users for longer than 5 years was increased by 30-40%. In women aged between 60 and 64 the increase rose to 70% after 5 years.

Prior to this, the "powers that be" touted HRT not just for youthfulness and for relief of menopausal symptoms but also for prevention of heart disease, incontinence, Alzheimer's disease, osteoporosis, and many others.

One by one, these supposed benefits have been disproved and, at present, the only recommended use for HRT is for the relief of hot flushes; and for a maximum of 5 years.

As we shall see, it is not specifically the oestrogen that can cause problems but also the progestins and/or the combination of the two. Again, we must point out that many of these ERT and HRT products are not the natural hormone. They are the synthetic similar product made by drug companies so that the product can be patented.

If, in the beginning, natural, bio-identical hormones were used, and prescribed on an individualised basis, giving physiological replacement, then possibly many of the problems may never have occurred.

Perhaps I should ask a general question … *Where do we get our information from?*

Information comes from a variety of sources. There are books and there are medical journals, and there is the internet. The internet is full of the good, the bad and the ugly. Sometimes it is difficult to tell the difference.

A major source of information for many doctors is directly from the drug companies. Is this a good source?

I don't believe it is. The companies that provide doctors with information are biased towards their own products. This results in a conflict of interest.

Medical journals *should* be a good source of correct information, but are they?

The *New York Times* (4 August 2009) published an article titled, **Medical Papers by Ghostwriters Pushed Therapy.**

"Newly unveiled court documents show that ghost-writers paid by a pharmaceutical company played a major role in producing 26 scientific papers backing the use of hormone replacement therapy in women, suggesting that the level of hidden industry influence on medical literature is broader than previously known. The articles, published in medical journals between 1998 and 2005, emphasized the benefits and de-emphasized the risks of taking hormones to protect against maladies like aging skin, heart disease and dementia. That supposed medical consensus benefited Wyeth*, the pharmaceutical company that paid a medical communications firm to draft the papers, as sales of its hormone drugs, called Premarin and Prempro, soared to nearly $2 billion in 2001."

"The ghost-written papers were typically review articles, in which an author weighs a large body of medical research and offers a bottom-line judgment about how to treat a particular ailment. The articles appeared in 18 medical journals, including The American Journal of Obstetrics and Gynecology and The International Journal of Cardiology. The articles did not disclose Wyeth's role in initiating and paying for the work. Elsevier, the publisher of some of the journals, said it was disturbed by the allegations of ghost-writing and would investigate. The documents on ghost-writing were uncovered by lawyers suing Wyeth and were made public after a request in court from PLoS Medicine, a medical journal from the Public Library of Science, and The New York Times."

<u>Note</u>* Wyeth - A Multi-National Drug Company, the manufacturer of these products.

This is a frightening trend. How can we believe what we read?

We must look closely at what we read and ask ourselves a few questions.

"Who wrote the paper?"

"Who would benefit from this?"

"Who paid for the research?"

Dr Peter Baratosy MBBS FACNEM

"Are there any conflicts of interest?"

Dr Eva Snead (1992), in her book, 'Some Call it AIDS... I Call it Murder,' gave six guidelines for determining accuracy.

1) When any issue becomes the object of media hoopla and financially lucrative, be on guard.

2) If an article is first published in an obscure foreign magazine, the information is probably correct.

3) If harmful data are published by those who may get hurt by their disclosure, the data is probably correct.

4) If a study set out to "demonstrate" something, this is not science but marketing. This does not mean you cannot learn from it. Read it thoroughly as their lies and denials tell you more than their affirmations.

5) A study financed by grants from a government agency or drug or chemical company is automatically suspect.

6) Above all, you cannot have it both ways at the same time: consistency and substance must be your guide.

It is important to scrutinize all that we read, which would include this book as well!

So, who do we believe?

From a philosophical point of view, natural, as designed by nature, must be right.

Natural, bio-identical oestrogen and progesterone are much safer than synthetic HRT.

How do we know?

First and foremost, it makes sense that the hormone, which is an exact copy of the hormone that the human body makes and uses, is safe and appropriate.

I must add that any substance, natural or otherwise, can be dangerous in *inappropriate* doses. The philosophy of using natural hormones is to replace with a dose that reflects what the normal physiological levels would be in the body (physiological dosage). This is much easier to do with natural hormones that are made by compounding pharmacists because doses can be individually adjusted.

Synthetic HRT comes in fixed doses; and the premise that you shouldn't worry if your needs do not fit exactly into the fixed dose.

Women do not come in standard sizes and therefore do not necessarily fit standard size doses of hormones.

49

There were very limited studies done prior to 2002. However, after the release of the WHI, and the increasing popularity of natural hormones, more research has been done, which has largely shown that the natural is better and safer than the synthetic.

When finally, a synthetic versus natural HRT study was done, the natural was shown to be definitely safer than the synthetic. The following section will discuss many of these studies.

In January 2009, a local paper, the *Adelaide Advertiser*, published an article about a new contraceptive pill being trialled in Sydney. The comment was made that this pill *"will revolutionise the lives of two million Australian women."*

This new miracle pill that had everyone talking was using the natural form of oestrogen called oestradiol.

"Finally," I thought, when I read the article, "they are seeing the light." I hoped that they would realise that they also needed to use the natural progesterone in order to have a much safer product.

Eventually, micronised progesterone capsules were introduced and became available on prescription as of 1 September 2016. This product is not, however, on the Pharmaceutical Benefits Scheme (PBS), and therefore is not subsidised by the government. There are advertisements in various medical journals where it is referred to as a "body-identical" hormone!

Remember the quote from Schopenhauer!

"All truth passes through three stages. First, it is ridiculed. Second, it is violently opposed. Third, it is accepted as being self-evident."

It is interesting to note that HRT is now called MRT–menopausal replacement therapy. HRT seems to have become a dirty word–so they changed the name!

The big problem with oral hormones is that after absorption, the hormone goes straight to the liver for metabolism–the "first pass effect"–a large amount is metabolised. Therefore, a larger oral dose needs to be given to achieve an appropriate dose in the body after the liver deals with it.

New studies show that the natural hormone is safer than the synthetic and point to the use of the synthetic progestin as the main reason for the safety issue.

Fournier, Berrino, Riboli, Avenel, and Clavel-

Chapelon (2005) showed that the rate of breast cancer was significantly higher in the women using synthetic progestin compared with the group using micronised progesterone. Micronised progesterone is an oral form of natural progesterone. The use of synthetic progestins, even in the short term, was associated with a significantly increased risk for breast cancer.

Olsson, Ingvar, and Bladström (2003) showed an increased risk of breast cancer in the group of women using oestradiol with progestin compared with oestradiol alone.

The main risk seems to be the use of progestins, such as medroxyprogesterone acetate (MPA). So, the questions to ask are, *"Are all progestins the same?"* and *"Is it just MPA, or is it all progestins?"*

Fournier, Berrino, and Clavel-Chapelon (2008) released a comparison study of breast cancer risks associated with different hormone replacement therapies. They posited that *"Large numbers of hormone replacement therapies (HRTs) are available for the treatment of menopausal symptoms. It is still unclear whether some are more deleterious than others regarding breast cancer risk."*

The researchers compared:

1) "never users" of HRT", with

2) oestrogen only users, with
3) oestrogen and progestin users, and finally, with
4) oestrogen and progesterone users.

The researchers found that compared with the "never users", the oestrogen users' risk was raised but the oestrogen-progestin users had the highest risk. The lowest risk was the oestrogen-progesterone users.

They also found that it did not matter which progestin was used, they were all much the same, i.e. bad. The researchers concluded that the choice of progestin was important, and it would be preferable to use progesterone (i.e. the "real thing")

In another study:

"The potential for an increased risk of breast cancer linked to the use of synthetic progestins combined with oral estrogens is one of the main putative reasons for discouraging postmenopausal women from using any type of hormone replacement therapy (HRT) for more than a few years. The hypothesis of progesterone decreasing the proliferative effect of estradiol in the postmenopausal breast remains highly plausible" (de Lignières, 2002).

> Real natural progesterone should be used–it is much safer.

You may ask why the choice of progesterone is important. The simple answer is because the synthetic form causes more damage and side effects. In many of the cases of problems with HRT, for example those highlighted by the WHI study, it appears that the use of progestin may have caused the problems.

The use of un-opposed oestrogen has been shown to cause an endometrial cancer, so a progestogenic agent *had* to be added to the mixture to protect the lining of the uterus. This, in some ways, was a good and a bad move. The use of a substance to balance the oestrogen to protect the uterus from cancer was a good move, but the choice of a synthetic progestin was not a good move.

As already mentioned, and as I will further explore, the synthetic progestin is probably what causes most of the problems. If natural progesterone had been chosen to balance the oestrogen, then many of the issues may not have occurred.

The WHI study showed that women on HRT,

meaning a combined oestrogen (generally horse derived oestrogens) combined with a synthetic progestin (MPA or similar), increased the incidence of heart attacks, strokes, blood clots, breast cancer and dementia.

Thomas, Rhodin, Clark, and Garces (2003) used a new technique: fluorescence imaging. This allows video microscopic recordings of blood flow, blood vessel morphology and blood cell activity in a live animal. They showed that synthetic progestin caused endothelial disruption, accumulation of monocytes in the vessel wall, platelet activation and clot formation. All these can lead to atherosclerosis, inflammation, and thrombosis.

This did not happen with progesterone, or with oestrogens.

Many of the side effects found from HRT in the WHI may have been due to the progestin alone.

Fournier, Mesrine, Boutron-Ruault, and Clavel-Chapelon (2009) looked at breast cancer and its relationship to HRT commencement at menopause. The results showed increased breast cancer in those who used HRT even for short periods (less than 2 years) if HRT was commenced close to menopause. This increased risk was *not* seen in hormone replacement containing progesterone.

Does oestrogen cause cancer?

Oestrogen does cause cancer; this has been well known for a long time. Oestrogen was put on the US National Toxicology Programme officially as a carcinogen in 2002, not just as a "possible carcinogen" but as a *"known* carcinogen" (Nelson, 2002).

However, some studies have shown that oestrogen does not cause cancer and may even provide protection.

One key point should be highlighted; oestrogen, out of proportion to progesterone, is dangerous. Oestrogen in balance with progesterone is safer.

Anderson et al. (2004) wrote that *"The use of CEE increases the risk of stroke, decreases the risk of hip fracture, and does not affect CHD (coronary heart disease) incidence in postmenopausal women with prior hysterectomy over an average of 6.8 years. A possible reduction in breast cancer risk requires further investigation. The burden of incident disease events was equivalent in the CEE and placebo groups, indicating no overall benefit. Thus, CEE should not be recommended for chronic disease prevention in postmenopausal women."*

A sub-group of 10,739 women, from the WHI study, were randomised to CEE or placebo groups.

Stefanick et al. (2006) concluded that *"Treatment with CEE alone for 7.1 years does not increase breast cancer incidence in postmenopausal women with prior hysterectomy."*

However, after one year, 9.2% of the women in the CEE group had abnormalities in the mammogram compared to only 5.5% in the placebo group and this pattern continued throughout the trial. There were more mammographic abnormalities in the CEE group compared with the placebo group. However, the authors state that this difference was primarily in assessments requiring short interval follow up. It is unclear what the authors meant by this, but possibly the CEE group had more benign breast abnormalities that needed investigations.

In this study, women who had undergone a hysterectomy were looked at as a separate category. As there was no uterus to develop endometrial cancer, those who had a hysterectomy could be treated with oestrogen only. This also led to the idea that hysterectomised women did not need to take progestogens.

Rock et al. (2008) wrote, *"Epidemiologic studies fairly consistently show in postmenopausal women that reproductive steroid hormones contribute to primary breast cancer risk, and this association is strongly supported by experimental studies using laboratory animals and model systems."*

The researchers continued *".... results from this study provide evidence that higher serum estrogen concentration contributes to risk for recurrence in women diagnosed with early-stage breast cancer."*

What is going on?

How do we explain this paradox?

How can we explain that a known carcinogen given to women does not cause breast cancer and may even provide protection?

The term "oestrogen" is not specific because oestrogen refers to a class of molecules, not to one specific molecule (contrast *progesterone*, which is one specific molecule). Humans have three major oestrogens: oestradiol, oestrone and oestriol.

First, we must differentiate between natural oestrogen, synthetic oestrogen and other substances that have oestrogenic activity, the so-called xenoestrogens. Thousands of chemicals have been introduced into our environment that have an oestrogenic action. These include pesticides, herbicides, phthalates (found in cosmetics), and polyvinyl chlorides (PVC, found in plastics), petrol and diesel exhausts, and factory emissions. These chemicals have infiltrated the air we breathe, the water we drink and the food we eat. We are living in a sea of oestrogen. Groundwater is contaminated with these chemicals; a large part is the residues of synthetic oestrogens coming from the urine of hundreds of thousands of women who take these synthetic hormonal products.

These oestrogens are polluting our environment and are having a disturbing effect on wildlife as well as on humans.

Oestrogens in the groundwater, in the rivers and lakes, are having a devastating effect on the wildlife. Frogs and fish have been shown to have the distinction between male and female blurred. As well as the damage they are doing to our animals and our environment, these xenoestrogens in our environment are contributing to a host of health problems in humans, including obesity, diabetes, early puberty, breast cancer, endometriosis, fibroids, miscarriage, low sperm counts and testicular cancer. I highly recommend that you read the book 'Our Stolen Future' by Colborn, Dumanoski, and Myers (1996).

This, of course, alludes to the fact that we, of all in the history of mankind, are exposed to the greatest number of oestrogens ever known. Up until 100 years ago, the only oestrogens that our bodies had to deal with were:

1) endogenous (i.e. made by the body) and

2) phytoestrogens, from the diet.

Now we are exposed to a huge number of exogenous (from outside the body) oestrogens (xenoestrogens = foreign oestrogens).

It is this total burden we must look at.

Next, we must look at the potency. Synthetic oestrogens, CEE (horse's oestrogen) are much more potent than human oestrogen and they attach to the receptors more strongly than the natural hormone, therefore prolonging stimulation. Also, the synthetic and "other species" hormones can block the effect of the natural hormones by occupying the receptor sites.

Finally, we should look at the way the oestrogens are metabolised. Hormones in the body, whether endogenous or exogenous, must be metabolised by the liver. The liver has the job of detoxifying the body by altering oestrogenic molecules and excreting them. The purpose of detoxification is to make a molecule less active and more water soluble, so it can be excreted more easily.

Oestrogen can be metabolised along three major detoxification pathways (the good, the bad and the ugly!), forming end products; 2 hydroxy oestrone, 4 hydroxy oestrone, and 16 hydroxy oestrone. Two of these end products (4 hydroxy and 16 hydroxy oestrone) have been shown to be *more* oestrogenic than the mother hormone and to be carcinogenic. On the other hand, 2 hydroxy oestrone has much less oestrogenic action and is not carcinogenic. In fact, it is the opposite, cancer protective.

Kabat et al. (1997) have shown that measuring 2 hydroxy to 16 hydroxy ratios can be predictive of breast cancer development. An elevated 2/16 hydroxy ratio can be predictive of breast cancer.

Eliassen, Missmer, Tworoger, and Hankinson (2008) showed that this ratio is more significant for oestrogen receptor negative, progesterone receptor negative tumours.

While Arslan et al. (2014) showed that *"higher levels of 2-OHE1(2 hydroxy oestrone) were associated with reduced risk of ER+ breast cancer in postmenopausal women after adjustment for circulating estrone."*

To protect ourselves from cancer, we must promote oestrogen metabolism down the 2 hydroxy pathway. How we do this is discussed in the treatment section of this book.

Earlier we saw that oestriol comprises the largest

percentage of oestrogen (60-80%) while the other two comprise only 10-20%. Since all three oestrogens compete with each other for the oestrogen receptor site, a high oestriol will compete with the much more potent oestradiol for binding and reduce the oestrogenic action of the more potent oestrogen. We have also seen that the CEE (horse's urine) has a high percentage of equilin, a much more potent oestrogen than human oestrogen and a high percentage of oestrone, the in-between potent oestrogen. All this adds up to a more potent oestrogenic stimulation which can be carcinogenic.

Oestriol is the oestrogen of pregnancy and is known to be breast protective. During pregnancy, when the breast cells are dividing in preparation for lactation, oestriol is high (so is progesterone), which would have a protective effect.

- Oestriol has the least stimulating effect on the breast.
- Oestradiol is possibly the most stimulating.
- Oestrone is in between.

Again, we must highlight the importance of good liver function. The liver is one of the most metabolically active organs in the body. One of its main jobs is to detoxify and remove metabolic wastes, by-products, and other substances. If the liver is compromised, or just over-loaded, then its efficiency declines. Remember, the liver was designed for, and evolved in, a much cleaner environment. Now it has a much greater burden to handle.

The liver can also be affected by metabolic syndrome (MetS). MetS does affect liver function and encourages cancer development. This will be discussed in the treatment section. See also my previous book 'Death by Civilization' (ISBN 978-0-6451053-7-7).

The liver detoxifies through two phases: Phase 1 and Phase 2. Phase 1 consists of the cytochrome P450 enzymes which utilise the process of oxidation, reduction, or hydrolysis to begin the process.

Phase 2 continues the detoxification by a process known as conjugation. The products generated by Phase 1 are coupled (conjugated) to various amino acids (glycine, glucuronic acid and the sulphur containing amino acids: cystine, taurine and methionine) or to the peptide glutathione. Oestrogen conjugates preferentially to glucuronic acid, and these oestrogen-glucuronide conjugates end up in the gut via bile for excretion.

However, there are bacteria in the gut that "love" glucuronide. These bacteria secrete an enzyme called *beta glucuronidase,* which breaks this conjugate bond. The bacteria then absorb and use up the glucuronide and leaves free oestrogen in the gut. The body absorbs and re-cycles this oestrogen. The result is that the body has not excreted any oestrogen. Again, dealing with this issue will be discussed in the treatment section of this book.

So, in summary, it is not just the oestrogen *per se* that must be considered; it is also

1) the type of oestrogen,
2) the total oestrogenic burden, the addition of endogenous and exogenous oestrogens, and
3) the way our body handles the oestrogen.

Hormones work generally in pairs; one tends to compliment yet antagonise the other. A great analogy is the car. Have you ever seen a car with just an accelerator, or just a brake? No, of course not. A car needs both an accelerator and a brake to achieve fine control.

It is the same with hormones. Oestrogen is the accelerator, it makes things grow, but there also needs to be a brake, which is progesterone, the real thing not the synthetic, not the counterfeit.

At this present moment, since oestrogens have been classified as a known carcinogen, it is best to avoid them. The exception would be where there is a deficiency state, the judicious use of an appropriate physiological replacement dose, in conjunction with real progesterone.

Breast cancer

Progesterone protects against breast cancer.

Chang, Lee, Linares-Cruz, Fournier, and de Ligniéres (1995) performed a study where various combinations of creams were rubbed onto the breast prior to surgery for non-malignant breast tumours. The women were allocated to groups receiving:

1) placebo,
2) oestrogen,
3) progesterone, and
4) oestrogen and progesterone.

Samples of breast tissues were examined for cell division. The number of cell divisions was greater in the oestrogen cream group, the lowest number was in the progesterone group. The oestrogen/progesterone group was in-between.

Progestins may cause breast cancer.

Fabre et al. (2008) wrote that *"The premenopausal use of progestogens (progestins) after the age of 40 years may be preferentially associated with the risk of lobular breast cancer and differentially affect the risk of breast cancer according to the hormone receptor status."*

65

Progesterone has a significant impact on breast cancer. Mohr, Wang, Gregory, Richards, and Fentiman (1996) performed an interesting study, where the researchers looked at the timing of breast cancer surgery. They found that if surgery for breast cancer was performed during the luteal phase of the cycle, i.e. when the progesterone level was high, there was an improvement in prognosis.

Singhal et al. (2016) showed the benefit of progesterone in breast cancer. *"Use of progesterone for treatment of breast cancer has raised considerable controversy because of past studies showing some negative effects of synthetic versions of progesterone used in hormonal therapy for postmenopausal women. In our studies, we are using natural progesterone, or forms of this hormone that are biologically identical to the natural hormone and testing it on breast cancer tissue taken from women with cancer."* (Emphasis the author.)

We can look at this at the molecular level.

Genes have been found to promote cancer and to inhibit cancer growth.

The length of cell life is regulated: one factor tries to keep the cell living longer and the other causes it to die off quickly. This planned cell suicide is called *apoptosis.*

One gene designated as p53 controls the rate of *apoptosis.* Another gene, called Bcl-2, is a gene that blocks apoptosis. Again, these two genes need to work together, like a brake and accelerator. Obviously, if the brake is out of action, things will grow faster.

Progesterone has been shown to down-regulate the Bcl-2 gene, which increases apoptosis in breast cancer cells (Formby & Wiley, 1998).

Progesterone has also been shown to increase apoptosis in ovarian cancer by up- regulating p53 gene (Bu et al., 1997).

While we are talking about genes, many may have heard about the cancer genes that occur in some families. These are the BRCA-1 and BRCA-2 genes. These are *normal* genes. Everyone has them. These genes make a protein that is involved in DNA repair. They are an important part of our protection from DNA damage that leads to cancer.

The problem in these families is that there is a mutation of the BRCA-1 and BRCA-2 gene. This mutation makes a protein that does *not* repair the DNA and therefore does not protect against cancer. Therefore, the people with this mutated gene tend to develop more cancer.

67

As we have already seen, there was a reduction in breast cancer, especially in the over 50-year-olds. This drop started in 2003 after the WHI report was released. This reduction was due to hundreds of thousands of women stopping the synthetic HRT (Katalinic & Rawal, 2008).

Ravdin et al. (2007) concurred.

WHAT ELSE IS HRT SUPPOSED TO DO?

We were told that HRT will protect the heart, prevent urinary incontinence, and prevent Alzheimer's or other dementias and prevent osteoporosis.

Now let's look at the truth.

Myth 1: HRT protects against heart disease

Many years ago, the opinion was that oestrogen protected women from heart disease. After all, the incidence of heart disease was low in younger women and did rise after menopause, when the levels of oestrogen fell.

This is another reason, they concluded, that men have heart disease because they do not have the "benefit" of oestrogen protecting them. They were so sure of this that in 1973, researchers put men on oestrogen to prevent heart disease. They were astounded that the men actually developed more heart attacks (The Coronary Drug

Project, 1973).

We now know this to be wrong. Oestrogen (on its own) is the culprit. Testosterone is the protective factor. Physiological replacement of testosterone is cardio-protective in women (Rako, 1998).

As a woman ages, the oestrogen levels drop, but so does the level of testosterone. It is the reduction in testosterone that is one of the triggers of heart disease (Debing et al., 2007).

Testosterone is the protective factor in heart disease. Low levels can cause heart disease. Debing et al. (2008) showed *"a positive association between low serum androgen levels and severe ICA atherosclerosis in men. It suggests that higher but physiological levels of androgens could have a protective role in the development of atherosclerosis."*

As a comparison, if we look at body builders, many have used testosterone and have developed heart disease. In that situation, be aware that they are using synthetic testosterone in excessive, supra-physiological doses.

Physiological replacement of the natural hormone is safe and beneficial: supra-physiological supplementation with synthetics is dangerous.

There are increased death rates in chronic heart failure in men with low levels of hormones. Researchers looked at the three hormones;

1) dehydroepiandrosterone (DHEA),
2) testosterone, and
3) insulin-like growth factor-1 (IGF-1).

The researchers found a 27% 3-year survival rate if *all* three hormones were low. If only two hormones were low, there was a 55% 3-year survival rate, a 74% 3-year survival rate with deficiency in only one hormone and an 83% 3-year survival rate if no hormones were deficient (Jankowska et al., 2006).

Since it was originally thought that oestrogen was heart protective, HRT was given to women for the purpose of protecting their heart, no matter if there were no menopausal symptoms, no matter if there was no heart disease. This was given because the women were in "the right age group". This was considered a "plus" as it was suggested that not only would women be "protected" from the menopause, but their heart would also be "protected".

We now know this to be false.

HRT can *cause* heart disease.

The Heart and Estrogen/Progestin Replacement

Study (HERS) was the first study to examine the effect of HRT on women with heart disease (Hulley et al., 1998).

The result of the study was "surprising" to the researchers, as they expected the study would show protection. However, the study showed that oestrogen plus progestin in post-menopausal women with heart disease did *not* prevent further heart attacks or death from coronary heart disease. Moreover, HRT increased the risk of clots in veins (deep vein thrombosis (DVT)), and lungs (pulmonary embolus).

As part of the WHI study, there was a relation between HRT and heart disease. Women on HRT developed more heart disease than women on the placebo.

"Estrogen plus progestin does not confer cardiac protection and may increase the risk of CHD among generally healthy postmenopausal women. Especially during the first year after the initiation of hormone use. This treatment should not be prescribed for the prevention of cardiovascular disease." (Manson et al., 2003). (Emphasis the author.)

Here again, it could be that the heart problem was caused by the choice of progestin. In contrast, progesterone, the real thing, has shown to be heart protective by *"preventing microvascular cardiac ischaemia"* (Hermsmeyer, Thompson, Pohost, & Kaski, 2008).

I do not generally support animal studies, and their relationship to human disease may not be valid. However, I will mention one experiment where Rhesus monkeys were used. The researchers were looking at coronary artery vascular spasm as a cause of death from heart disease. They induced vascular spasm in the monkeys using pathophysiological stimulation without injury. The monkeys on medroxyprogesterone and oestradiol went into vascular spasm and would have died if no intervention was given. The monkeys on progesterone and oestradiol did not go into vascular spasm (Miyagawa, Rösch, Stanczyk, & Hermsmeyer, 1997).

The PEPI (Postmenopausal Estrogen/Progestin Intervention) trial was implemented to *"assess pair-wise differences between placebo, unopposed estrogen, and each of three estrogen/progestin regimens on selected heart disease risk factors in healthy postmenopausal women."*

The participants were randomly assigned into 5 groups:

1) Placebo,

2) Conjugated equine estrogen (horse's urine) CEE,
3) CEE plus cyclic medroxyprogesterone acetate (MPA),
4) CEE plus continuous MPA, or
5) CEE plus micronised progesterone.

The endpoints of the study looked at HDL-C cholesterol, systolic blood pressure, serum insulin and fibrinogen.

The researchers concluded that *"Estrogen alone or in combination with a progestin improves lipoproteins and lowers fibrinogen levels without detectable effects on post-challenge insulin or blood pressure. Unopposed estrogen is the optimal regimen for elevation of HDL-C, but the high rate of endometrial hyperplasia restricts use to women without a uterus. In women with a uterus, CEE with cyclic MP [micronized progesterone] has the most favorable effect on HDL-C and no excess risk of endometrial hyperplasia"* (The Writing Group for the PEPI Trial, 1995).

This is one study that *did* use the real thing: progesterone. The results show that progesterone is safe and effective as compared to the synthetic progestin.

It is unfortunate that the WHI study did not include a progesterone group.

Myth 1 BUSTED.

Myth 2: HRT protects against urinary incontinence

Urinary incontinence (UI) is defined as uncontrollable, involuntary leaking of urine, and is a problem for many women. In the early days, HRT was recommended to treat incontinence. The thinking was that oestrogen protected the vagina and surrounding tissues and this, theoretically, should support the bladder and thus prevent incontinence.

I should point out here that the vagina is an oestrogen dependant tissue; topical oestrogen is an excellent treatment for an atrophic, dry vagina.

This was initially made on an assumption. Women were put on HRT to treat and even prevent incontinence. However, research later found that HRT not only did *not* help the problem, but actually caused it to be worse.

When further results from the HERS study were analysed, Steinauer et al. (2005) found that women with a history of heart disease who were in the group that did *not* have UI at baseline and who took HRT, had a significantly increased rate of UI.

This needed more research.

Hendrix et al. (2005) wrote, *"Menopausal hormone therapy has long been credited with many benefits beyond the indications of relieving hot flashes, night sweats, and vaginal dryness, and it is often prescribed to treat urinary incontinence (UI)."* Women were randomised, depending on hysterectomy status, to either placebo, oestrogen only or oestrogen with progestin (CEE + MPA).

The researchers concluded that *"Menopausal hormone therapy increased the incidence of all types of UI at one year among women who were continent at baseline."* They also noted that *"Conjugated equine estrogen with or without progestin should not be prescribed for the prevention or relief of UI."*

Anecdotally, this does not seem to happen with natural, bio-identical hormones.

In fact, there is evidence that it is not the female hormone but the male hormone, testosterone, that can be beneficial for women with UI. Yes, testosterone, the "male" hormone.

Ho, Bhatia, and Bhasin (2004) showed that *"Androgens induce muscle hypertrophy and reduce fat mass. The action of androgens in the lower urinary tract and pelvic floor is complex and may depend on their anabolic effects, hormonal modulation, receptor expression, interaction with nitric oxide synthase, or a combination of these effects. Further studies are needed to determine the precise role of androgens in women with urinary incontinence and pelvic organ prolapse."*

Two studies have been done that show oestrogen and testosterone have a positive effect on UI. However, note that these experiments were done on rats (Cayan et al., 2008; Madeiro et al., 2002).

Certainly, from an anecdotal, clinical perspective, I have been treating women with UI with a low percentage testosterone cream, applied directly to the vagina/urethra area with very positive results.

Myth 2 BUSTED.

Myth 3: HRT protects against Alzheimer's disease and dementia

We have seen that HRT was once recommended for prevention of dementia and Alzheimer's disease (AD). Women were put on HRT to keep not only their bodies healthy but to keep their mind sharp. So far, we have seen that HRT possibly did more harm than good.

Since AD affects twice as many women as men, oestrogen could be the reason. In a study, 42 women with mild-to-moderate AD were assigned to either placebo or CEE. After 16 weeks, there was no difference (Henderson et al., 2000).

In the same edition of the same journal, another study looked at the same thing. Fifty women with AD were randomised to either placebo or CEE. The study only ran for twelve weeks and after that time, there was no difference between the two groups (Wang et al., 2000).

These two studies were too short and had too few participants.

A longer study with more women needed to be done.

A total of 120 women with mild-to-moderate AD were randomised to either a placebo, low dose of CEE, or a higher dose of CEE. After one year, there was little difference, with perhaps a slight worsening on the Clinical Dementia Rating Scale among the women on CEE (Mulnard et al., 2000).

The conclusion was that oestrogen, well, at least horse's oestrogen, does not have a role in treating AD. Perhaps it made it worse.

The role of prevention was not explored.

A study called WHIMS (Women's Health Initiative Memory Study) looked at a sub-set (approximately 3,000) of the women in the WHI study. They ranged from ages 65-79 and were either on placebo, CEE, or CEE with MPA. The researchers were looking for signs of AD or other forms of mental or memory decline. The results showed that the HRT did not reduce the incidence of AD or mental decline.

What was even more concerning was that the women over 65 years who were on HRT, on average, had a greater decline in overall mental function than those who took the placebo. The researchers concluded that *"Use of hormone therapy to prevent dementia or cognitive decline in women 65 years of age or older is not recommended"* (Shumaker et al., 2004).

It gets even worse!

Resnick et al. (2009) showed that not only does HRT increase dementia, but it makes the brain shrink. This finding was based on brain MRI scans of 1,403 women, aged 71-89 years, who were participants in the WHIMS study. The women were either on placebo, CEE, or CEE with MPA.

The results showed greater brain atrophy in women with either combination of hormones, compared with placebo. Women on HRT had a 2.37 cubic centimetre reduction of brain volume, especially in the frontal lobe, which is responsible for memory and thinking skills.

The researchers concluded that *"Conjugated equine estrogens with or without MPA are associated with greater brain atrophy among women aged 65 years and older; however, the adverse effects are most evident in women experiencing cognitive deficits before initiating hormone therapy."*

The original theory was that "mini strokes" caused the memory and thinking problems. However, this research was done on women where MRI brain scans showed that the underlying cause was NOT "mini strokes" but brain atrophy (shrinkage).

Why was it first thought that HRT could protect women against dementia? Was it because fewer women on HRT developed dementia?

There certainly may be a bias.

Observational trials are biased, mainly because it is generally the healthier women that are on the HRT. This is what is known as the "Healthy User Bias Effect" leading to the incorrect belief that HRT prevented dementia (or heart disease, or whatever) when, in reality, the women were healthier from the start.

Here again, it could be the progestin that caused the problem, not necessarily the oestrogen.

So, the studies that have been done indicate that HRT not only does not prevent AD, but may even aggravate it.

What about natural hormones?

I mention this because anecdotally, women who seem to be suffering from dementia do become mentally brighter when started on progesterone. This is an observation that many practitioners have noted.

Unfortunately, there are no studies that look at progesterone and AD.

Carrol et al. (2007) used oestrogen and progesterone in special transgenic mice, which is an animal model of AD.

> It should be noted that translating the results of animal experiments to human diseases is controversial and may not necessarily be valid.

The researchers found that oestrogen and not progesterone prevented the accumulation of the beta-amyloid, which is a feature of AD. When oestrogen and progesterone were given together, then the progesterone *"blocked the beneficial effect* of oestrogen."

However, on a more positive note, the researchers noted that, *"... progesterone significantly reduced tau hyper-phosphorylation when administered alone or in combination with oestrogen. These results demonstrate that oestrogen and progesterone independently and interactively regulate AD-like neuropathy and suggest that an optimised hormone therapy may be useful in reducing the risk of AD in postmenopausal women. "*

As discussed, synthetic hormones, especially progestins, do not prevent and may even cause AD, so we should explore whether the natural hormones can protect. Progesterone is known to be neuroprotective. Could it be that the reduced level of progesterone, especially in women, can contribute to AD?

A review by Singh and Su (2013) emphasized the difference between progesterone and MPA (hence the negative results in the WHIMS study), as well as suggesting that the reduced level of progesterone with ageing could contribute to AD. They also comment on the fact that progesterone is neuroprotective.

Yoon et al. (2018) found that *"Long-term MHT (Menopausal Hormone Therapy) using percutaneous E2 (Oestradiol) gel and oral MP4 (Micronised Progesterone) might attenuate cognitive decline in postmenopausal women with MCI (Mild Cognitive Impairment)."*

Note that these women were also on *donezepil*; an anti-cholinesterase inhibitor used to treat AD. The hormone group was compared to a placebo group, i.e. both groups were on the drug.

How effective is donezepil? The medication does help some, but overall has only minimal effect.

"Treatment of dementia with cholinesterase inhibitors and memantine (another AD drug) *can result in statistically significant but clinically marginal*

improvement in measures of cognition and global assessment of dementia" (Raina et al., 2008).

"Donepezil is not cost effective, with benefits below minimally relevant thresholds. More effective treatments than cholinesterase inhibitors are needed for Alzheimer's disease" (Courtney et al., 2004).

"There is moderate-quality evidence that people with mild, moderate or severe dementia due to Alzheimer's disease treated for periods of 12 or 24 weeks with donepezil experience small benefits in cognitive function, activities of daily living and clinician-rated global clinical state" (Birks & Harvey, 2018).

AD is a multi-factorial condition and there is no one single drug that is optimal for treatment.

Many practitioners who use bio-identical hormones, which include progesterone, have observed mental improvement in elderly women on starting B-HRT.

How can we explain this?

Perhaps we should look at it from another angle.

Why should progesterone do positive things to the brain?

First, we do know that there are progesterone receptors (PR) in the brain (Brinton et al., 2008).

Then the question to ask is, *"If there are such receptors in the brain, what function do they have?"*

We do know that the risk for AD is higher in women than men, so perhaps there is a hormonal connection. Many studies have looked at oestrogen, however, it is important to recognise that progesterone also falls precipitously during menopause.

Progesterone has been shown to be neuro-protective, although the exact mechanism is still not fully known (Kaur et al., 2007).

There is growing evidence that progesterone has a neuro-protective effect on the central nervous system (CNS). Studies have shown that the administration of large doses of progesterone (NOTE: progesterone *not* progestin) during the first few hours to days after brain injury limits CNS damage, reduces loss of neural tissue and improves functional recovery. The published research focuses on blunt traumatic brain injuries, however, there is evidence that progesterone can protect the brain from acute CNS injury, including penetrating brain trauma, stroke, anoxic brain injury and spinal cord injury.

"Progesterone appears to exert its protective

85

effects by protecting or rebuilding the blood-brain barrier, decreasing development of cerebral edema, down-regulating the inflammatory cascade, and limiting cellular necrosis and apoptosis. All are plausible mechanisms of neuroprotection" (Stein, Wright, & Kellermann, 2008).

Note: this does not happen if progestins are used.

Schumacher, Guennoun, Stein, and De Nicola (2007) showed that progesterone can be synthesised by neurons and glial cells within the nervous system.

"...there is growing evidence that this hormone (progesterone) may be a safe and effective treatment for traumatic brain injury and other neural disorders in humans" (Stein, 2008).

Here we can speculate.

Progestins cause more harm. MPA has many CNS side effects. Could it be that the MPA, which has a shape and structure like progesterone, has a *blocking* effect on the PR, which prevents progesterone from doing its usual job?

Could the reason why MPA and other progestins are causing so many adverse effects is because they block the PR and prevent progesterone from doing what it normally does?

From a clinical point of view, progesterone does *not* have the usual good positive effects if taken together with a progestin.

Progestins possibly are progesterone receptor blockers.

Myth 3 BUSTED

Myth 4: HRT protects against osteoporosis

Osteoporosis is a bone disease that occurs when the body loses too much bone, makes too little bone, or both. As a result, bones become weak and may fracture from a fall, or in extreme cases, even from minor trauma, e.g. sneezing or minor bumps.

(https://www.bonehealthandosteoporosis.org/patients/what-is-osteoporosis/ accessed 23 April 2024)

To understand osteoporosis, it helps to look at the mechanism of normal bone formation. Bones are continually being made and un-made. The overall balance of the two processes determines whether bone is strong or osteoporotic. There are two main types of bone-forming cells: *osteoclasts* and *osteoblasts.*

Osteoclasts move through the bone and seek out and dissolve old bone. The second type of cell, osteoblasts move in and make new bone.

Osteoclasts are largely regulated by oestrogen. A decline in the level of oestrogen increases the activity of these cells and therefore increases the rate of bone breakdown. On the other hand, osteoblasts are largely regulated by progesterone. A deficiency of progesterone slows down bone production. So, bone breakdown exceeds bone production, and the result is osteoporosis.

Since osteoporosis was observed mainly in menopausal women, the connection was surmised as an oestrogen deficiency. Therefore, replacing oestrogen may improve the situation, because oestrogen *reduces* bone breakdown. However, it does not build it up. The mainstream medical profession was quite happy to add osteoporosis to the list of positive benefits of HRT.

Osteoporosis is not necessarily a condition of menopause. Some women have already lost a large percentage of bone even before they reach menopause, so whatever is causing it, it is not the supposed oestrogen lack. If women are having regular periods, then there is definitely no lack of oestrogen.

Why are these women osteoporotic if their oestrogen levels are normal?

Perhaps it is not the oestrogen, and therefore, other hormones should be considered.

Dr Jerilynn Prior, from the University of British Colombia, studied fit, healthy, non-menstruating female athletes (over-training can suppress periods) and found them to be osteoporotic. She also studied women, other than athletes, and noted that many had anovulatory cycles (Prior, Vigna, Schechter, & Burgess, 1990).

No ovulation = no progesterone.

The similarity in both cases was a *lack* of progesterone. Her research showed that oestrogen has only a minor role in bone formation, while progesterone has a much more important function.

Prior (2018) showed that *"clinically normal cycles commonly have ovulatory disturbances (anovulation, short luteal phases) and low P4* (progesterone) *levels; these are more frequent in teen and perimenopausal women and increased by everyday stressors: energy insufficiency, emotional/social/economic threats and illness."*

Prior, Naess, Langhammer, and Forsmo (2015)

showed that *"Anovulation in a random population occurs in over a third of clinically normal menstrual cycles."*

If a woman does not ovulate, then a corpus luteum does not form, and therefore does not make progesterone. These women are progesterone deficient.

The use of progesterone cream in the treatment of osteoporosis has only been a recent development, which was pioneered by Dr John R. Lee. In his book, he describes his experiences using progesterone cream in the treatment of osteoporosis.

He treated women with proven osteoporosis, as measured with bone densitometry. In a relatively short time, significant rises in bone density occurred (Lee, 1991).

Prior (2018) concurred that progesterone is beneficial in building bone.

Case Study

I was treating a 70-year-old lady with osteoporosis with progesterone cream. She went for her regular follow up bone densitometry and afterwards, she told me that they repeated the test a few times because the results showed a dramatic increase in bone density. They thought their machine was not calibrated properly. They had not seen such a dramatic increase in bone density before.

So, it is the progesterone, not the oestrogen.

Of course, mainstream practitioners had difficulty accepting this. Many excuses were made, mainly that progesterone cream does not absorb (note: now most hormone replacement is given via a transdermal route, the hormone patch or gel) and it is dangerous because the uterus may not be protected.

In the following discussion, we will see that these points have been refuted.

Another arm of the PEPI trial looked at the effects of hormone therapy on bone mineral density.

The participants were randomly assigned into five groups:

1) Placebo,
2) Conjugated equine estrogen (Horse's urine) CEE,
3) CEE plus cyclic medroxyprogesterone acetate (MPA),
4) CEE plus continuous MPA, or
5) 5/) CEE plus micronised progesterone.

Results, not unexpectedly, showed a decline in bone density in the placebo group.

Those in the active groups gained bone density, although there was not that much difference among the four active groups (The Writing Group for the PEPI., 1996).

The important point is that the treatment of osteoporosis is *long term*. We have seen previously that the use of HRT in the long term may be dangerous.

Since osteoporosis needs *long term treatment*, logically, the *safest* treatment should be chosen, and that would be progesterone.

Riis, Thomsen, Strøm, and Christiansen (1987) studied 57 women who were divided into two groups: placebo and active. The active group was given transdermal oestradiol, then after a year, cyclic progesterone was added for another two years. The placebo group continued just on placebo cream. The women were assessed regularly. There was a significant decrease in bone density in the placebo group (not unexpected). In the active group, bone density remained constant and was not influenced by the addition of the progesterone.

Of course, progesterone is not the choice of drug companies; they prefer to use their patented, similar, synthetic hormone.

Does the progestin MPA have the same positive benefit?

No!

Prior et al. (1997) compared CEE (horse's oestrogen) with MPA. Women were divided into two groups: one group was on CEE and the other group on MPA. They were followed up for one year with regular bone densitometry and blood tests.

Bone loss was prevented by the CEE, but not the MPA. It is a shame that they did not include a group of women on progesterone.

So, CEE can prevent osteoporosis (remember that oestrogen prevents bone breakdown) BUT remember also that the use of unopposed oestrogen is dangerous as it can cause a uterine cancer.

In another study, Prior, Vigna, Barr, Rexworthy, and Lentle (1994) used cyclic MPA. This study showed bone density increases with MPA.

However, I reiterate that treatment of osteoporosis is a long-term prospect. Although MPA did increase bone density, the long-term side effects, as we have seen earlier, possibly would cause more harm than good.

93

Oestrogen prevents bone breakdown.
Progesterone builds up bone.

Lydeking-Olsen, Beck-Jensen, Setchell, and Holm-Jensen (2004) looked at isoflavone containing soymilk and compared that with transdermal progesterone.

"Given concerns over the use of hormone replacement therapy (HRT), women are seeking natural alternatives to cope with the symptoms and effects of menopause. The bone sparing effects of soy protein and its isoflavones are well established in animal studies, while 5 previous human studies on soy and bone have yielded variable outcomes due in part to their short duration of study. Progesterone has been suggested as a bone-trophic hormone, but the effect of long-term, low dose transdermal progesterone is unknown."

This group of women was divided into four treatment groups:

1) Soymilk containing isoflavinoids,
2) Transdermal progesterone,
3) Soymilk plus transdermal progesterone, or

4) Placebo (isoflavone poor soymilk and progesterone free cream).

Here again, there was not unexpected bone loss in
the placebo group.

There was no bone loss in the soymilk group or in
the transdermal progesterone group. However, there was
bone loss in the soymilk plus transdermal progesterone
group. The reason for this was not explained.

Unfortunately, there are only a few studies done on
progesterone in the treatment of osteoporosis. This
possibly boils down to money and profit. Why spend
millions of dollars on a substance you cannot patent?

Up to this point, another hormone has not been
mentioned in the context of osteoporosis, and that is
testosterone.

Yes - the male hormone.

What does this have to do with osteoporosis, which
occurs more frequently in women?

Women do make testosterone, however, only
about one tenth of that made by males. Yet even that
small amount is necessary.

Testosterone is certainly well known to have a muscle and bone building effect on the body. A deficiency of testosterone in some menopausal women may play a part in the development of osteoporosis.

Women *can* become testosterone deficient; symptoms include unexplained fatigue, lack of wellbeing, and diminished libido. Of course, many of these symptoms are generalised and can only be diagnosed if the woman's testosterone level is measured. Unfortunately for many women, their doctor does not know this, and so does not consider testosterone deficiency when looking for a cause of the above symptoms.

The use of testosterone in women is becoming more widespread and possibly can be used as a prevention and treatment of osteoporosis.

Many years ago, nandrolone (Deca-Durabolin), an injectable form of synthetic testosterone, was a recommended treatment for osteoporosis in menopausal women.

This product is still used today, although not as the first line treatment. The recommendation is to use only where other therapies have failed.

The supplementation of testosterone is especially important for women who have had a total hysterectomy, i.e. removal of womb and both ovaries (Davis, 1999).

Testosterone should never be given alone but in conjunction with other hormones, preferably bio-identical.

Of course, as I have said many times, the hormones that need to be replaced should be replaced by bio-identical hormones, and in physiological doses, to achieve a physiological level.

This is important because excess testosterone in a woman could cause side effects of masculinization, such as hirsutism (excess body hair growth), deep voice and clitoral enlargement.

Another androgen that has been shown to have positive benefits in women is dehydroepiandrosterone (DHEA).

DHEA is a steroid hormone, produced mainly by the adrenal glands and is the precursor for both testosterone and oestrogen. The level of this hormone declines with age. Villareal, Holloszy, and Kohrt (2000) showed that supplementation of this hormone can give positive benefits. Men and women with low DHEA levels can partially reverse the age-related changes in fat mass, fat-free mass, and bone mineral density.

von   Mühlen,   Laughlin,   Kritz-Silverstein,

Bergstrom, and Bettencourt (2008) concluded that *"Among older healthy adults, daily administration of 50 mg of DHEA has a modest and selective beneficial effect on BMD and bone resorption in women, but provides no bone benefit for men."*

Some have raised concerns that supplementing testosterone in women could cause breast cancer.

Dimitrakakis, Jones, Liu, and Bondy (2004) showed no increase in breast cancer with the addition of testosterone. In fact, the researchers commented that there may even be a protective factor.

Bitzer, J., Kenemans, P., Mueck, A.; for the FSDeducation Group. (2008) did a literature search looking at breast cancer and testosterone. They concluded that *"... there are no valid randomised or observational clinical studies that provide evidence that the addition of testosterone to conventional postmenopausal hormone therapy influences breast cancer risk."*

Myth 4 partly busted.

There is an opinion held by many that women who

have had a hysterectomy do not need to take progesterone. This idea seems to be based on the notion that progesterone only influences the uterus.

This is *not* correct.

Progesterone receptors are known to exist in hormone sensitive tissues such as breast and uterus, however they have been found in many other, non-hormone sensitive tissues, including:

- bladder (Rizk, Raaschou, Mason, & Berg, 2001),
- aortic endothelium (Welter, Hansen, Saner, Wei, & Price, (2003),
- thyroid (Money et al., 1989),
- brain (Brinton et al., 2008) and
- bone (MacNamara, O'Shaughnessy, Manduca, & Loughrey, 1995).

Progesterone receptors must have some function in these tissues. Consider what has already been discussed, that there are progesterone receptors in the artery, brain, bladder, bone–all tissues that have been mentioned above where HRT has been shown to have a negative effect. Could it possibly be that the progestins are acting as progesterone receptor blockers and preventing progesterone from carrying out its normal function?

Progestins have a similar shape and structure, and

they attach to the progesterone receptor. However, unlike a lock and a key, the attachment is not perfect.

What else do the experts tell us?

Many self-styled experts state that natural hormones do not work, that the natural hormone creams do not absorb through the skin.

This is curious, because, today, most of the drug company synthetic hormones are given transdermally by a patch or cream. I would assume they work as they have been approved by the relevant authorities.

The term "expert" is often overused these days, and it is helpful to ask:

Who are they working for?

Who is paying them to say these things?

I will let you, the reader, decide for yourself.

According to the "experts", natural hormones do not work. It is odd that they would suddenly stop working after humanity survived for countless generations, with only natural hormones.

Ask any woman who is on natural hormones -

preferably prescribed by someone who is trained and gives appropriate doses. She will more than likely give a glowing report about how well she feels.

I have seen many women that were miserable on synthetic HRT. They made the decision to change to B-HRT and they are glad they did.

So, do bio-identical hormones work, or is it that the women using them are deluding themselves?

One prominent study published in the *Medical Journal of Australia* (Wren, 2005) made the headlines. The study describes the use of transdermal progesterone, and it showed no benefit. The tone of this research is one of negativity.

As we have seen, synthetic hormones can cause many negative side effects. However, this study has been quoted many times to "prove" that progesterone cream does not work. The conclusion seems to say that natural progesterone cream does not work, so go back to the synthetics! This conclusion flies in the face of clinical experience.

Since the release of the WHI study, many women are too scared to go on synthetic HRT and wish to use the natural hormone, generally as a cream.

Clinically, they do get benefit, but only if

prescribed by appropriately trained doctors giving appropriate doses.

New studies have now been done that show that the cream actually does work.

Burry, Patton, and Hermsmeyer (1999) showed that transdermal progesterone cream is absorbed well. *"The percutaneous application of progesterone cream appears to be a safe and effective route of administration."* However, there were only six women in the study, and it lasted for only four weeks.

L'hermite, Simoncini, Fuller, and Genazzani (2008) wrote that *"... the transdermal route of administration of estrogens and the use of natural progesterone might offer significant benefits and added safety."*

Vashisht, Wadsworth, Carey, Carey, and Studd (2005) looked at transdermal progesterone in conjunction with transdermal oestrogen. Serum levels of progesterone and oestrogen were significantly elevated, although the levels were low. However, the women reported *"significant reductions in menopausal symptoms." "Natural progesterone creams are gaining popularity as a possible treatment for menopausal symptoms, and many women may be using them with estrogen. We planned to evaluate, using an open plan study, the systemic absorption of a combination of transdermal estrogen and progesterone. Women applied transdermal progesterone 40 mg and transdermal estrogen 1 mg daily over 48 weeks. Women were assessed at intervals of 12 weeks. Significant increases in plasma levels of progesterone and estradiol were seen after 12 weeks, although only low plasma progesterone levels were found (median 2.5 nmol/l) and no further increase was noted over the remainder of the study period. A significant correlation was found between plasma levels of the two hormones (r = 0.315, p = 0.045). Women reported significant reductions in menopausal symptoms, as measured by the Green Climacteric Scale, after 24 and 48 weeks of combined treatment. There may be similar mechanisms of absorption of the two hormones, although the doses used in our study produced sub-luteal levels of progesterone. There was no evidence of accumulation of progesterone with time, and further study is needed to assess the efficacy and safety of this combination of hormones."*

Previously, in the USA, progesterone was available in over the counter (OTC) cosmetic creams; it is a wonderful moisturiser. I think it is worth pointing out that this progesterone cream had been an OTC product for a very long time and no dangers had been shown.

Hermann et al. (2005) were concerned that this

unregulated topical cream could have risks. Their study showed that transdermal progesterone cream produced similar blood levels as oral micronised progesterone capsules. I do agree with the authors in some ways; however, I do not share their worry about the dangers, although I agree that progesterone should be monitored and prescribed by appropriately trained professionals.

In many studies, progesterone is measured as a "serum level". This may be inaccurate as progesterone in a fat-soluble molecule and, as we all know, oil and water do not mix. This last study was done on whole blood.

Koefoed and Brahm (1994) showed that a large proportion of steroid sex hormones, including progesterone, circulates in the blood bound to the cell membranes of the red blood cell (RBC). Just measuring the watery part of the blood can give an inaccurate reading.

Another two studies have shown the safety and effectiveness of bio-identical hormones.

"Physiological data and clinical outcomes demonstrate that bioidentical hormones are associated with lower risks, including the risk of breast cancer and cardiovascular disease, and are more efficacious than their synthetic and animal-derived counterparts"

(Holtorf, 2009).

"The studies reviewed suggest bioidentical progesterone does not have a negative effect on blood lipids or vasculature as do many synthetic progestins, and may carry less risk with respect to breast cancer incidence. Studies of both bioidentical estrogens and progesterone suggest a reduced risk of blood clots compared to non-bioidentical preparations" (Moskowitz, 2006).

Topical progesterone cream does absorb adequately and has been shown to be safe.

A major criticism of transdermal progesterone by the mainstream is the fear that endometrial hyperplasia caused by the oestrogen is not dealt with adequately by the lack of action of the transdermal progesterone.

This concern has now been answered.

Leonetti, Landes, Steinberg, and Anasti (2005) compared a group of women on CEE and MPA with a group of women on CEE and transdermal progesterone. The women had endometrial biopsies before, during, and after. The results showed that 77% of the women preferred the CEE with transdermal progesterone. There was no endometrial hyperplasia in any group. The researchers concluded that CEE with transdermal progesterone has a similar action on the endometrium as standard HRT.

The mainstream keeps telling us that these natural hormones are dangerous and cause all sorts of side effects. So far, we have seen that the natural hormones are safe - very much safer than the synthetic.

Stephenson et al. (2004) showed that the transdermal cream worked and did not have side effects, which the synthetics did. We know that the synthetics cause blood clots, so this study looked, not only at menopausal symptom relief from a transdermal progesterone but also at various haematological parameters. Using the Green Climacteric Scale, the researchers showed that the women rated their symptoms on the progesterone cream as "significantly improved". Also monitored were various blood parameters: factor VII:C, factor VIIa, fibrinogen, antithrombin, PAI-1, CRP, TNF and IL-6. All remained unchanged. The researchers concluded that progesterone cream relieves menopausal symptoms without adversely effecting bleeding and clotting, which can be a problem with conventional HRT.

What we have here is a conflict between drug

companies trying to sell their synthetic hormones, and the women of the world who are resisting because of the studies that show the synthetics are more dangerous and the natural is safer.

Medical education

Mainstream doctors only know about synthetic HRT. This is what they are taught in medical school, read about in the journals, see in the drug advertisements, and are informed about by the drug representatives that visit on a regular basis.

Unfortunately, they do not know anything else. This reminds me of the saying, *"When all you have is a hammer, everything looks like a nail."*

Since there is a lot of money in pharmaceutical products and a large amount of pharmaceutical money is invested in medical teaching, it is no wonder that the natural B-HRT is not emphasised. In fact, just the opposite occurs; B-HRT is actively vilified.

It is interesting to note, however, that over the last 5-10 years, major pharmaceutical companies are starting to use natural hormones and using a transdermal route.

Remember the quote from Schopenhauer? *"All*

truth passes through three stages. First, it is ridiculed. Second, it is violently opposed. Third, it is accepted as being self-evident."

I have often stated the importance of any product, whether natural or not, being in the correct dose. Even a natural product, such as a herb, a vitamin, or a mineral, can be dangerous in inappropriately high doses, or ineffective in low doses.

However, the *window of safety* is much broader for a natural product than for a pharmaceutical drug. Natural is definitely much safer.

> Physiological replacement for
> physiological deficiency.

Although HRT use has been the subject of many studies, these have been primarily for marketing purposes rather than science.

For many years, HRT was recommended for heart disease prevention, for osteoporosis prevention, for bladder incontinence prevention, for Alzheimer's prevention; for keeping young in general. Newer studies have disproved most of these.

At present, the only use for HRT is for the prevention of hot flushes and then for only a maximum of 5 years, as after this time, negative effects begin.

TESTOSTERONE

Testosterone has developed a bad reputation.

This very useful, and essential, hormone has been lumped together with anabolic steroids that are being used by athletes and bodybuilders to gain more strength and more muscle bulk.

Although testosterone is generally associated with men and masculinity, it is also a critical hormone for women.

The bad reputation developed because it was being abused in high, supra-physiological doses, which, as well as being illegal, is considered cheating in the sporting arena. The authorities are trying to keep sport "clean," anabolic steroid enhancement free. As with many other drugs that are not legal, the sale of these drugs has gone underground. With the market now an illegal one, there is no quality control of the products, which may be smuggled in from other countries, or produced locally in clandestine laboratories. Either way, quality control is poor. There is no way of knowing what you are injecting or swallowing!

We know that these substances are being used in large quantities. As far back as 1995, illegal steroids represented a $US1 billion black-market trade (Hoberman & Yesalis, 1995).

Even more worrying is the recent development of "designer steroids", which are drugs designed to be undetectable using current drug testing methods. These substances have not been fully researched. Many "designer steroids" must stay one step ahead of the testing authorities.

You may find it hard to believe, but research is limited, confused and contradictory. There is a lot we do not know. Investigation is difficult because of the secretive nature of usage; many are reluctant to divulge their use and be involved in medical research. The research conducted is based on self-confessed users, yet precise details of the doses used are not known for sure.

Even before we look at testosterone use, there is the issue of the use of *synthetic* testosterone analogues, such as methyltestosterone, oxandrolone, oxymetholone and nandrolone. These are the preparations mainly used by abusers who inject or ingest these substances, usually in massive doses, to achieve a physical increase in muscle bulk, strength, and increased performance.

The damage that occurs could either be due to the huge doses used or because of the adverse effects of the synthetic testosterone. Also, we must not forget that the people using these hormones are generally fit and healthy and, presumably, have normal testosterone levels.

These substances are not testosterone, but are similar. As with oestrogen and progesterone, the synthetic testosterones can cause more side effects.

Natural testosterone taken orally is well absorbed but due to the "first pass effect"; anything absorbed through the stomach goes straight to the liver and five-sixths is broken down to inactive metabolites. This means that only one sixth of the dose remains as the active testosterone. To overcome this, testosterone was modified. A methyl group was attached at the 17 position and became methyltestosterone. This is active orally and is not metabolised by the liver. This product, however, is not used very much today due to liver toxicity problems (Westaby, Ogle, Paradinas, Randell, & Murray-Lyon, 1977).

Testosterone can also be esterised (either as a propionate, enanthate, undecanoate or cypionate) which can then be administered by injection. Once injected, an enzyme breaks the ester bond and releases free testosterone. These substances are oily, and this allows the testosterone to be released slowly. Injection seems to be the most common method for non-medical usage.

Androgenic-anabolic steroids (AAS) have two major properties: They promote male characteristics, and they also have anabolic features, which is the ability to promote protein development which increases muscle bulk.

Testosterone has an androgenic/anabolic ratio of 1:1. Different synthetic testosterone analogues have different ratios. This is important, as men more often want more anabolic features and less androgenic features. In women, there should be hardly any androgenic features.

Androgenic/anabolic ratios are determined by animal experiments; however, this does not necessarily translate to the human population.

The men who use these products are generally fit and healthy younger men who want to increase their bulk, strength, and performance. Presumedly, these men have normal testosterone levels; if so, how appropriate is the supplementation of even more?

The use of high supra-physiological doses in young healthy men may be dangerous and lead to long term ill health.

Hartgens and Kuipers (2004) wrote, *"Androgenic-anabolic steroids (AAS) are synthetic derivatives of the male hormone testosterone. They can exert strong effects on the human body that may be beneficial for athletic performance. A review of the literature revealed that most laboratory studies did not investigate the actual doses of AAS currently abused in the field. Therefore, those studies may not reflect the actual (adverse) effects of steroids."*

They also noted that *"The main untoward effects of short- and long-term AAS abuse that male athletes most often self-report are an increase in sexual drive, the occurrence of acne vulgaris, increased body hair and increment of aggressive behaviour. AAS administration will disturb the regular endogenous production of testosterone and gonadotrophins that may persist for months after drug withdrawal. Cardiovascular risk factors may undergo deleterious alterations, including elevation of blood pressure and depression of serum high-density lipoprotein (HDL)-, HDL2- and HDL3-cholesterol levels. In echocardiographic studies in male athletes, AAS did not seem to affect cardiac structure and function, although in animal studies these drugs have been observed to exert hazardous effects on heart structure and function."*

Many case studies have been published in journals on the deleterious use of anabolic steroids.

"Manifestations of severe coronary artery disease after anabolic drug abuse" (Mewis, Spyridopoulos, Kühlkamp, & Seipel,1996).

"Acute myocardial infarction in a young man using anabolic steroids" (Wysoczanski, Rachko, & Bergmann, 2008).

"An acute myocardial infarction occurring in an anabolic steroid user" (Huie,1994).

"Ischemic stroke related to anabolic abuse" (Santamarina, Besocke, Romano, Ioli, & Gonorazky, 2008).

The trouble with these papers is that they are case studies, each reporting on just one patient.

There are some adverse things we do know.

High dose androgenic-anabolic steroids *do* reduce HDL (the "good" cholesterol) and increase the LDL (the "bad" cholesterol) thus increasing the possible risk for coronary artery disease (Hurley et al., 1984).

Graham et al. (2006) showed that prolonged use (over 20 years) of AAS increases homocysteine levels, which increases the risk for future thromboembolic events.

One concern is the increase in heart muscle thickness. Anabolic steroids bulk up muscle, so it can also bulk up the heart muscle. A bulky heart can pump harder - up to a point. However, when it becomes too bulky, function can deteriorate.

Some studies have investigated the hearts of bodybuilders who have used anabolic steroids.

Dickerman, Schaller, Zachariah, and McConathy (1997) concluded that *"Anabolic steroids may potentiate concentric left ventricular hypertrophy with decreasing ventricular compliance without affecting cardiac function."*

Dickerman, Schaller, and McConathy (1998) showed that *"Retrospectively, 43% of the drug-free bodybuilders and 100% of the steroid users had left ventricular wall thickness beyond the normal range of 11 mm."*

They also noted that *"The use of anabolic steroids concomitant with intensive resistance exercise does appear to augment left ventricular size without dysfunction."*

Salke, Rowland, and Burke (1985) compared

117

bodybuilders using steroids, and bodybuilders not using steroids with an inactive control group. They found thickened heart muscle in the body builders, but there was no relation to steroid usage.

Could it be that the heart muscle thickening is due to the heavy exercise workload these men do?

As you can see, various studies have differing results, so ultimately, there is little conclusive data, although there seem to be more studies that show heart wall enlargement than not.

What about long-term use and damage?

D'Andrea et al. (2007) looked at AAS use. The researchers found ventricular wall thickness in both the AAS users and non-users. In this study, they specifically looked at ex-long-term users, i.e. those that had stopped using AAS for 5 years. They again found ventricular wall thickening similar in both ex-users and non-users and this was thicker than a group of sedentary controls. They concluded that *"Several years after chronic misuse of AAS, power athletes show a subclinical impairment of both systolic and diastolic myocardial function strongly associated with mean dosage and duration of AAS use."*

Urhausen, Albers, and Kindermann (2004) showed long-term damage with AAS use. They concluded that *"Several years after discontinuation of anabolic steroid abuse, strength athletes still show a slight concentric left ventricular hypertrophy in comparison with AAS-free strength athletes."*

Other dangers,

- AAS use reduces sperm production, causes shrinking of the testes, impotence, difficulty and/or pain on urination, baldness and irreversible breast enlargement (gynecomastia).
- Females who use AAS develop more masculine traits, decreased body fat, decreased breast size, deepening of the voice, increase in body hair and clitoral enlargement.
- AAS use in teenagers of both sexes can stop the adolescent growth spurt so that they end up with a shorter stature.
- AAS users of either sex can develop liver abnormalities, blood clotting abnormalities, hypertension, and cholesterol changes; that can lead to heart disease and stroke.
- AAS use may lead to more aggressive behaviour, the so called "roid rage."
- Depression, fatigue, restlessness, loss of appetite, insomnia, reduced libido, headaches and aches and pains in joints and muscles can develop on *stopping* AAS.
- The black-market supply of these substances of dubious quality and the sharing of needles can lead to infections, such as HIV, hepatitis B and C, septicaemia, abscesses, and so on.

119

Steroid use has long-term effects.

The knowledge of the use of anabolic-androgenic steroids has increased. This is not to say it is right, but usage today is perhaps better, definitely smarter, than in the past.

Previously these drugs, of unknown source and quality were used indiscriminately and in doses unknown. Today, the usage is on a more cyclical basis. This may be for safety reasons, although it is more than likely to avoid the routine drug testing regimes the sports authorities have instigated to catch drug cheats.

Physiological replacement in men and women

Testosterone should be reserved for the population of men and women, who have signs and symptoms of testosterone deficiency, and who have been shown to have low levels. They can be supplemented, in appropriate physiological doses, to achieve physiological normal levels. This would also imply continual monitoring with appropriate tests.

Physiological replacement is the very
important concept here.

As you have seen, the use of high dose, synthetic testosterone analogues *can* cause damage. What about the "proper use" of these substances? There is ample evidence to show that physiological replacement is safe and has none of the problems as discussed above.

Many doctors are afraid of prescribing this hormone. It could be that they are concerned about doing so because of the controversy over athletes, body builders and hormone use. As well, there is a great deal of misinformation about the dangers and usefulness of testosterone.

However, many studies have shown testosterone to be beneficial in appropriate doses, and in the appropriate population.

Testosterone replacement therapy (TRT)

Testosterone replacement implies that there is a deficiency, and that this deficiency is treated by giving adequate replacement. This applies to women as well as men. In contrast, giving large doses of hormone to someone whose levels are normal, just so they can run faster or grow bigger muscles is inappropriate, and in my opinion, wrong.

In the right situation, replacing testosterone in men

and women can be lifesaving. Of course, we cannot live forever.

Replacing hormones is not necessarily aimed at prolonging life. Rather, the aim is to improve quality of life, making those remaining years more pleasant with improved energy, improved vigour and reduced degeneration of mind and body.

> The use of testosterone in physiological replacement doses, in men and women, is safe.

As a man or woman ages, the levels of testosterone and other hormones decline, and this has an effect. Some may regard this as normal ageing, a part of life. Others look at it from another perspective. If low levels of hormones cause symptoms and disease and normal levels prevent degeneration, then why not supplement these hormones to "normal" levels and lead a more pleasant life?

Have a look at the symptoms of low testosterone. Some of these symptoms are similar in both sexes and are non-specific. They may be related to ageing, but are they ageing itself?

Symptoms of low testosterone in men.

* Loss of libido

* Erectile dysfunction

* Fatigue

* Memory loss

* Loss of muscle mass

* Moodiness

* Irritability

* Poor motivation

* Joint aches and pains

* Hot flushes

* Poor sleep

> ## Symptoms of low testosterone in women
>
> *Loss of libido
>
> * Fatigue
>
> * Memory loss
>
> * Weakness
>
> * Moodiness
>
> * Poor motivation
>
> * Joint aches and pains
>
> * Poor sleep

A more philosophical question is - What is "normal" ageing?

What is a disease state?

There may be a fine line between these two.

More and more men and women do *not* accept these symptoms, and they do *not* accept that this may be related to "just getting old" and "ageing gracefully". They do not want to end up as "grumpy old men" or "grumpy old women". They want to be more pro-active.

Andropause

The term "andropause" is used to describe the male equivalent of menopause, yet it is a controversial concept. The first thing we must consider is, does it even exist?

There are some who deny that this condition exists at all. They argue that it is just a part of ageing.

The above symptoms are nonspecific and may be related to ageing, but I say that there is more to andropause than ageing. There are men who develop distressing symptoms, who, on investigation, are found to have low testosterone levels. These men can be supplemented with testosterone as a therapeutic trial, and many improve and achieve a better quality of life.

I argue that the men who get the above symptoms do so because of a decline in their testosterone levels. However, is the ageing a result of hormone decline, or is hormone decline a part of ageing?

Dr Peter Baratosy MBBS FACNEM

Interesting question.

Of course, not all men go through such a stage; some feel well and do not have any complaints. They may be the more confident ones, accepting the symptoms of ageing. Some of these are the healthy ones and cope well with ageing. They may have low testosterone levels but have no symptoms.

There is a population of men who do *not* accept the symptoms and want to do something about them.

Some equate andropause with hypogonadism; basically, low testosterone levels caused by the ageing testes.

Whatever you think, we cannot deny that there is a group of men who are severely impacted by symptoms that deny them a quality of life.

Call it andropause, call it hypogonadism, call it ADAM ("androgen deficiency of ageing male") or PADAM ("partial androgen decline in ageing males"). Call it what you like, these men need help.

If tests do show a low testosterone level, then a trial of testosterone replacement may be warranted. If it improves their quality of life, then isn't that worthwhile?

Female menopause is a bit more obvious. Treatment is, however, very different. Women were, for many years, put on HRT almost automatically, to either treat symptoms of moodiness and hot flushes, as well as to "prevent diseases", such as heart disease, osteoporosis, and so on, which we now know does not work. Some women were put on HRT based solely on their age.

Most doctors are men and, in the past, when they treated women, sometimes, they possibly over-treated them with a very paternal (and perhaps sexist) attitude. *"Don't worry your pretty little head about it ... just take these pills and you will be right."*

Although this attitude may not overtly present these days, the underlying sentiment still could be.

So why are men different? Why aren't men put automatically on hormones during the male menopause?

One reason is because it is under-recognised. Some doctors do not even believe it exists. Certainly, men do not complain as much and do not go to the doctor as readily as women.

Another reason is, again, that most doctors are males and somehow do not think men need hormone replacement.

The good news is that times and attitudes are changing.

Perhaps it is the "baby boomers" that want more out of life. They worked hard all their lives and now, in retirement, they want more. They will *not* accept that the tiredness, the irritability, the lessening of sexual function is "just a part of ageing".

They become more pro-active and demand something be done. The "baby boomers" are computer literate and search the 'net. They see that testosterone replacement could be the answer. If the doctor does not suggest it, then many men demand testosterone replacement. These men are informed and are armed with pages and pages of printed off material from the internet to show the doctor.

Cardiovascular disease

Many doctors feel uneasy about replacing testosterone because of the many myths that have been circulated.

For many years, testosterone was thought to be the culprit in heart disease; after all, more men than women had heart disease. However, it now seems that it is *not* the testosterone but the oestrogen. Higher oestrogen levels in younger men have been shown to increase heart disease. Tomaszewski et al. (2009) wrote that *"Increased levels of estrogens are associated with unfavourable lipid profile in men and this association is present early in life, before apparent manifestations of cardiovascular disease."*

As men age, their testosterone drops and the (relative) level of oestrogen increases. However, in women, as they age, oestrogen drops, but so does testosterone. It is the relatively higher oestrogen in relation to the lower level of testosterone that causes heart disease.

Tivesten et al. (2006) measured oestradiol in a group of men as well as carotid artery intima-media thickness. After three years, the researchers found that the men with higher oestradiol levels had worse thickening of the carotid artery. Carotid artery measurement is an indicator of overall arterial disease, which includes the coronary arteries.

Wranicz et al. (2005) showed that high oestrogen in men can cause heart disease.

The myth that testosterone causes heart disease is partly true, but this is when high doses of synthetic testosterone analogues are used by younger persons.

However, natural testosterone, in appropriate,

replacement doses, is safe and can protect against heart disease.

Heart disease is caused by a *lack* of testosterone in men (Nettleship, Jones, Channer, & Jones, 2009) and in women (Debing et al., 2007). Testosterone replacement can protect against heart disease in men and women.

Deenadayalu, White, Stallone, Gao, and Garcia (2001) showed that testosterone improves angina by inducing coronary artery dilation. This is achieved by opening the calcium-activated potassium channels, which relaxes the muscles in the coronary arteries.

English, Steeds, Jones, Diver, and Channer (2000) studied low dose transdermal testosterone in men and concluded that *"Low-dose supplemental testosterone treatment in men with chronic stable angina reduces exercise-induced myocardial ischemia."*

If testosterone can induce coronary artery dilation, can it also induce other arteries to dilate?

What about peripheral arterial disease (PAD)?

The ankle-brachial index (ABI), which reflects the state of arterial perfusion in the lower limbs, is a useful measure of peripheral vascular health. Serum free testosterone was positively associated with a good ABI, suggesting a vascular protective link, whereas free oestradiol was negatively associated with a good ABI (Tivesten et al., 2007).

Can supplementing testosterone to men with PAD improve symptoms?

Unfortunately, we do not know for sure, however, the evidence is suggestive that it can be beneficial.

A Cochrane study (Price & Leng, 2012) concluded that *"There is no evidence to date that short-term testosterone treatment is beneficial in subjects with lower limb atherosclerosis. However, this might reflect limited data rather than the lack of a real effect."* (Emphasis the author.)

As indicated above, testosterone is a vasodilator. Men who do have PAD must have some other form of artery disease and if symptoms fit, a trial of testosterone can only be beneficial.

What other arteries can testosterone dilate?

What about erectile dysfunction?

Since all arteries are connected and disease in one area can reflect disease elsewhere, erectile dysfunction (ED) can be viewed as an early indicator of systemic cardiovascular disease (Billups, Bank, Padma-Nathan, Katz, & Williams, 2005). Basically, if you can still have an erection, then your arteries in the rest of the body must still be in good working order.

Generally, erectile dysfunction (ED) is a vascular problem, not just a low testosterone problem. The damage to the artery may have already been done. This damage can be done by smoking, alcohol, pollution and/or by MetS. Hyperinsulinaemia causes vascular damage, and this can cause ED.

The MetS/hyperinsulinaemic patient is usually obese, diabetic, unfit, and hypertensive - all bad risk factors for the arteries.

Can testosterone have a vascular dilating effect on the penile artery?

Shabsign (2004) studied men with ED and low testosterone and who were *not* responsive to the drug sildenafil 100mg, i.e. Viagra, or the "little blue pill." The men were given testosterone replacement and the response to the drug was much improved.

Testosterone alone can improve erectile function in men with low testosterone levels. However, testosterone alone may not always be adequate due to the multifactorial nature of ED (Shabsigh, 2005).

The incidence of metabolic syndrome (MetS) in the western world is very high. According to Saklayen (2018) the incidence of MetS is about 25% of the world population, and this incidence will rise as the less developed nations adapt to a western-style diet and lifestyle.

As well as the health issues already mentioned, those with the syndrome have a higher risk of developing cancer. They also have a greater risk of developing arterial disease. A man with all these issues, who also has ED, will not necessarily respond to the use of sildenafil, or to replacing testosterone. These people need to change their diet and lifestyle; to get fitter, lose weight, eat better. They need to deal with the underlying metabolic problem, and this largely is related to the western diet and lifestyle. Many are on various medications, such as anti-hypertensive drugs and antidepressants, which are notorious for having ED as a side effect.

As an example, let's look at depression.

This is a very common problem. Depressed men are on anti-depressants: one of the side effects of these medications is ED. But then again, depressed men also have poor libido. Are these men low in testosterone and their depression is caused by low testosterone? Would it be more appropriate to treat these men who have low testosterone with testosterone replacement rather than an anti-depressant?

The bottom line is that in the treatment of ED, the person must be treated holistically.

Another fear is that testosterone will produce abnormal cholesterol levels. Certainly, high dose synthetics can do this, but too low levels also can. Correct levels of testosterone can normalise cholesterol levels.

As men age, testosterone levels decline and this is related to increasing levels of triglycerides and reducing levels of HDL, both being risk factors for heart disease (Zmuda et al., 1997).

Supplementing testosterone to men with low testosterone in physiological doses can reduce total cholesterol and reduce arterial inflammation by suppressing inflammatory markers (Malkin et al., 2004).

Cardiovascular (heart and artery) disease is thought to be mediated by inflammation.

Testosterone has been shown to reduce inflammatory markers and *"...may be important in inhibiting atheroma formation and progression to acute coronary syndrome"* (Malkin, Pugh, Jones, Jones, & Channer, 2003).

Increased death rates have been observed in chronic heart failure in men with low levels of hormones. Jankowska et al. (2006) looked at three hormones:

1) dehydroepiandrosterone (DHEA),
2) testosterone, and
3) insulin-like growth factor-1 (IGF-1).

The researchers found a 27% 3-year survival rate if all three hormones were low. If only two hormones were low, then there was a 55% 3-year survival rate, a 74% 3-year survival rate with deficiency in only one hormone, and an 83% 3-year survival rate if no hormones were deficient.

Prostate cancer

Another fear, or is it a myth, is that testosterone causes prostate cancer in older men?

Let's think about this for a while. When does prostate cancer develop? It develops in elderly men when the level of testosterone is the lowest! If testosterone is a cause of prostate cancer, then shouldn't it develop in young men when the levels are the highest?

This fear that testosterone may produce prostate cancer is preventing many men from receiving the benefits of testosterone replacement. Khera and Lipshuitz (2007) write that *"There are compelling data to suggest that testosterone replacement therapy (TRT) in normal and high-risk men does not increase the risk for prostate cancer."*

Morgentaler (2007) wrote, *"New evidence suggests that TRT has little, if any, negative impact on the prostate, even in men with a history of PCa (prostate cancer)."*

Testosterone alone does not cause prostate cancer.

So, what does cause prostate cancer? This is a hard question to answer, as there is no one solution. There are probably very many causes and reasons. One reason is oestrogen. Certainly, the environment is also important. There is the pollution, and there are the multitudes of toxic chemicals in the environment. Note that many of these pollutants have xenoestrogenic properties.

Other than the chemicals and pollution, the poor western diet must be considered; it is a highly refined, high-carbohydrate diet, which stimulates the increase in levels of insulin. This leads to hyperinsulinaemia and subsequent MetS. Cancer is one of the aspects of MetS.

Many doctors are reluctant to give testosterone to ageing males because of the fear of producing prostate cancer. Initially, this was based on a theoretical basis. When studies were done, there did not seem to be any relationship, yet the myth remained.

Prehn (1999) has even gone to the extent of saying that it is the *decline* in testosterone levels that contributes mostly to cancer development. Furthermore, supplementing testosterone may protect against cancer.

Hoffman, DeWolf, and Morgentaler (2000) maintain that there is an association of a low testosterone level with more aggressive and extensive prostate tumours.

There is a belief that replacing testosterone in men who have had prostate cancer is contra-indicated. The current dogma is that testosterone will cause the prostate cancer to grow even more out of control. *"Like throwing petrol on a fire!"*

This has turned out to be false.

Chedrawe, Sathe, White, Ory, and Ramasamy (2022) write *"Testosterone has since frequently been suggested to fuel PCa (prostate cancer). Researchers have since found that the relationship between androgens and PCa is more complicated, and likely not linear. For instance, men with the lowest levels of testosterone were found to be at an increased risk of biopsy proven PCa compared with other hypogonadal men. Furthermore, hypogonadal men who are on testosterone do not appear to have a higher risk of de novo PCa. And, in men with localized PCa and curative treatment, multiple studies have shown that giving testosterone therapy (TTh) does not appear to increase the risk of disease progression or recurrence."*

New research shows that in men with advanced prostate cancer and metastases, testosterone may not necessarily worsen the disease, although this is still being debated.

Morgentaler, Abello, and Bubley (2021) write *"These initial observations indicate TTh (testosterone therapy) was not associated with precipitous progression of PCa (prostate cancer) in men with BCR (biochemical recurrence) and MET (metastatic prostate cancer), suggesting a possible role for TTh in selected men with advanced PCa whose desire for improved quality of life is paramount."*

In men with no sign of prostate cancer, the possibility exists that it may influence the sub-clinical disease. For this reason, testosterone replacement should only be given to men once they have been adequately investigated and continual monitoring is recommended.

Marks et al. (2006) studied forty-four men, aged forty-four to seventy years, who were given either testosterone injections or placebo. Forty of the forty-four men had prostate biopsies at baseline and at the end of the study. No treatment-related change was found in the prostate biopsies.

The authors concluded that *"The prostate risks to men undergoing TRT (Testosterone Replacement Therapy) may not be as great as once believed, especially if the results of pre-treatment biopsy are negative."*

Rhoden and Morgentaler (2003) studied men proven by biopsy to have precancerous lesions and who were followed for one year on testosterone replacement. After one year of testosterone replacement, men with precancerous intraepithelial neoplasia (PIN) did *not* have a greater increase in PSA or significantly increased risk of cancer than men without the precancerous lesion.

There is little evidence that testosterone, on its own, causes prostate cancer.

So, what is it in the ageing male that can cause prostate cancer?

You may be surprised to hear that it is oestrogen.

Yes, oestrogen, the female hormone. Men do make some oestrogen and as the male ages, more oestrogen is produced, especially if there is obesity. This can readily be seen on the beach with elderly men developing "man boobs" / "moobs." The ageing testes make less testosterone, and there is a relative rise in oestrogen.

There is an enzyme called *aromatase,* which converts testosterone to oestrogen. *Aromatase* is found mainly in the fat cells. Obviously, if there are more fat cells, then there is more *aromatase.* This has the action of converting more testosterone to oestrogen; therefore, testosterone levels go down and oestrogen levels go up.

Oestrogen receptors are found in the prostate and with relatively higher oestrogen and relatively lower testosterone, Prins and Korach (2008) write that *"there is ample evidence through hormone-controlled studies and with in vitro approaches to clearly document that many of the estrogenic effects on the prostate are directly mediated through prostatic expression of estrogen receptors. "*

Aromatase can be inhibited. One of the main inhibitors is zinc. There is a high level of zinc deficiency in western society. With low zinc levels and more *aromatase,* it is no wonder that there is low testosterone and higher oestrogen in older men. Also, the increase in obesity is epidemic, which exacerbates the problem.

Obese men have more prostate cancer than thin men. This could party be due to the hyperinsulinaemia, causing increased growth factors, but it also could be due to the increased oestrogen.

Amling et al. (2001) showed that out of 860 men with advanced prostate cancer, 21% were classed as obese and 49% were classed as overweight. Obese patients were more likely to have a radical prostatectomy at a younger age, and a higher Gleason score (a staging score that classifies the extent and spread of cancer).

Another factor is the xenoestrogenic pollution. What is the effect of these hormone-mimicking pollutants on males? Ho, Tang, Belmonte de Frausto, and Prins (2006) showed that early exposure to these chemicals can predispose males to prostate cancer. This research was done in rats, so how much it relates to humans is not known for sure. It is a frightening prospect all the same.

Setlur et al. (2008) found a specific gene defect/mutation in about half of all prostate cancers. This defective gene acts as an on/off switch that is activated by oestrogen, giving the signal to multiply. These cancers tended to be the more aggressive ones that spread easily.

Oestrogen plays a role in the development of benign prostatic hypertrophy (BPH) and prostate cancer, although it may not be the only factor. It seems that both oestrogen and testosterone are involved.

On the other hand, progesterone seems to have a beneficial effect on the prostrate; not just on prostate cancer, but on BPH as well (Chen, Yu, & Dong, 2017; Kaore et al., 2012).

Diabetes and the metabolic syndrome (MetS)

I have mentioned metabolic syndrome (MetS) a few times already. This is a syndrome characterised by a cluster of conditions, the original four being diabetes, hypertension, obesity and high cholesterol. Cancer, Alzheimer's disease and many others can be added. See my previous book 'Death by Civilization' (ISBN 978-0-6451053-7-7), which looks at MetS in much more detail. The book can be ordered through any bookshop, or online.

The underlying metabolic abnormality is hyperinsulinaemia (too high insulin levels in the blood) with insulin receptor resistance developing. This means that there is plenty of insulin in the bloodstream, but the body does not respond because of the insulin resistance (IR). One of the ways this condition is treated is by improving IR with diet, exercise, and nutrients. Another way is to supplement testosterone.

Kapoor, Goodwin, Channer and Jones (2006) stated that *"Low levels of testosterone in men have been shown to be associated with type 2 diabetes, visceral adiposity, dyslipidaemia and metabolic syndrome."*

The authors continued, *"Testosterone replacement therapy reduces insulin resistance and improves glycaemic control in hypogonadal men with type 2 diabetes. Improvements in glycaemic control, insulin resistance, cholesterol and visceral adiposity together represent an overall reduction in cardiovascular risk."*

Is it the low testosterone that causes IR or does IR cause the low testosterone? It seems to be the latter. Pitteloud et al. (2005) have shown that IR influences the Leydig cells in the testes that make testosterone.

Low testosterone levels have been recognised as a reliable prognosticator of MetS. Spark (2007) suggests that testosterone replacement may be able to reverse some aspects of MetS.

Alzheimer's disease (AD)

In the previous section, we saw that women were put on (synthetic) HRT to prevent them from developing Alzheimer's disease (AD). However, research has shown the notion to be false. Not only does it *not* prevent AD, but it may also even make it worse!

We have discussed oestrogen and progesterone regarding AD, but what about testosterone?

Papasozomenos and Shanavas (2002) showed in a rat model that testosterone prevented hyperphosphorylation of tau. This is a technical term, which basically means that the protein which is thought to be important in AD is prevented from forming. These rat experiments showed that supplementing testosterone may prevent or delay AD in humans.

But how closely do rat experiments relate to humans?

Lu et al. (2006) studied men with mild AD who were compared with normal elderly controls. After 24 weeks, the researchers concluded that testosterone replacement therapy improved overall quality of life in patients with AD. Fuller, Tan, and Martins (2007) concurred.

The bottom line is that synthetic HRT does not help AD, and could make it even worse, however "real" testosterone (and progesterone) may be beneficial in AD.

Osteoporosis

In the previous section, we also looked at osteoporosis. Synthetic HRT was initially used to treat and to prevent osteoporosis, however, the results weren't good because of the long-term side effects.

Osteoporosis treatment needs to be long term, and the use of synthetic HRT long term has been shown to be hazardous.

Progesterone (the real thing) has been shown to have a positive action on bone. Testosterone has also been shown to have a positive effect, as it is an anabolic hormone, which is necessary to make the bones strong.

Osteoporosis has been shown to develop in men with low testosterone levels. Meier et al. (2008) concluded "... *serum testosterone is independently associated with the risk of osteoporotic fracture and its measurement may provide additional clinical information for the assessment of fracture risk in elderly men.*"

Testosterone supplementation has been shown to prevent and treat osteoporosis in men.

Testosterone can also be used in women for the treatment of osteoporosis. One important point to emphasize is that testosterone should never be given to women on its own. It should always be given together with natural, bio-identical progesterone, and plus or minus oestrogen.

Watts et al. (1995) studied surgically menopausal women who were randomly put on,

1) oestrogen or

2) oestrogen + androgen (Note: the form of androgen was methyltestosterone) and followed for two years.

At the end of two years, the researchers found that the treatments prevented bone loss in both groups, but the oestrogen + testosterone group was associated with a *"significant increase in spinal bone mineral density compared with baseline."* They also made the comment that the blood tests results had not changed, and therefore the combination was safe over the two years of treatment.

Davis, McCloud, Strauss, and Burger (1995) looked at oestrogen and testosterone implants in relationship to bone density and sexuality. The conclusion was that oestrogen and testosterone were better together than oestrogen alone for improving bone density. They also found that the combination had improved libido.

Libido

Libido can be defined as the basic ability to generate mental interest in sex. In other words, sexual desire.

In the male, this must be differentiated from erectile dysfunction (ED), which is the inability to achieve erection. If the man does not want to use the erection, that is a libido issue!

Libido in men and women is related to testosterone levels but is not the full story. Libido is a much more complex issue than just a hormone deficiency. It is a multifaceted interplay between the physical, the psychological, spiritual, and, importantly, includes relationship issues.

Why does libido go down?

Could it be simply biological? The desire for sex goes once the reproductive time has lapsed. This certainly happens in the animal kingdom.

Humans are more complex than that. Sexual activity in humans is more than just biology.

Why do humans lose their libido?

There are many reasons, only one of them being hormonal.

Below are some reasons for loss of libido:

- Chronic ill-health, such as MetS (which includes diabetes, vascular disease, obesity), hypothyroidism, etc.
- Drug use; illicit, or prescribed, alcohol problems, anti-depressants, anti-hypertensive medication, smoking, etc.
- Mental illness, such as depression.
- Relationship issues. "Loveless marriage."
- Health of partner.

All the above can interfere with libido and are probably not related to "hormones."

These issues need to be addressed. Giving testosterone before dealing with the above problems is a good reason why testosterone replacement does not work is all cases.

However, once these issues are sorted out and if there is still a libido issue, then hormonal help can be given.

Both men and women have the same hormones, but in different proportions. As the man or woman ages, the levels of sex hormones — oestrogen, progesterone, and testosterone — decline. Testosterone is considered the most important hormone as far as libido goes.

Ageing equals lower hormones.

Does ageing cause low hormones or do low hormones cause ageing?

This is a philosophical question.

Does it really matter? Some doctors certainly think so. They try to keep people younger by supplementing hormones to "youthful levels".

Libido declines with age. Libido and testosterone levels are strongly related at the population level but not necessarily on the individual basis (Travison, Morley, Araujo, O'Donnell, & McKinlay, 2006).

The issue can be complicated by individual factors in the individual person. There are men with low testosterone levels but who do not have ED or libido problems. The level of sexual activity in younger years can be a factor in libido in later years.

Men with chronic ill health may have normal testosterone levels but have a low libido.

In one study, 165 men with ED were assessed. Using total testosterone levels, only 4.8% were classified as hypogonadal. When using the "free" testosterone levels, 17.6% were classified as hypogonadal. There was no association between total and free testosterone levels and libido. When ED is more severe, it is more probable that "free" testosterone levels are below normal (Martínez-Jabaloyas, Queipo-Zaragozá, Pastor-Hernández, Gil-Salom, & Chuan-Nuez, 2006).

Just looking at testosterone levels is inadequate to make a full assessment. We must look at each person, and treat them holistically and as an individual, not just give them testosterone.

On the other hand, a trial of testosterone replacement in a person with low testosterone levels and low libido is a valid form of treatment.

Relationships can be a big factor. There are men who have ED and/or low libido with their wife, but not with their girlfriend!

Men and women with low libido have been shown to have low testosterone levels, although it is not the only factor. As a man or woman ages, the levels of hormones decline, as mentioned above. Ageing has been associated with decreased muscle mass, muscle strength, physical performance, physical activity, bone mineral density and libido. These non-specific clinical features may indicate organic testosterone deficiency.

For those in this age group with the above conditions, testosterone replacement may be of special importance (Wald, Meacham, Ross, & Niederberger, 2006).

Supplementing testosterone only to men with low libido and/or ED, as a part of treating andropause or male menopause, can improve libido. This may not occur in 100% of men but more than 50% will respond and although it could take 12-24 weeks to manifest (Yassin & Saad, 2007).

"Although a relatively small number of men with ED are found to have hypogonadism, sexual dysfunction is a common finding among all men with low testosterone. Administration of testosterone to men with hypogonadism and ED has been shown to bring about a significant improvement in their sexual function, energy,

mood and body composition" (Ojumu & Dobs, 2003).

Testosterone replacement is safe in the long term. One study followed men for two years with blood tests. *"Long term testosterone replacement to date appears to be a safe and effective means of treating hypogonadal elderly males, provided that frequent follow-up blood tests and examinations are performed"* (Hajjar, Kaiser, & Morley, 1997).

Monitoring is essential.

Elderly, hypogonadal men can be "grumpy old men"!

They have changes in mood, become angry and irritable, sad, tired, less friendly, and more nervous. Testosterone replacement in these men can improve mood. They become less angry and irritable, their energy improves, and they become more friendly and relaxed (Wang et al., 1996).

So, even if there is no increase in libido, they are much more pleasant to live with. This could be the extra bit that may improve the relationship with their spouse, which may then improve their sex life!

What about women?

As women age, their hormones decline.

Because of this, many women lose their libido, and this can lead to conflict and even marriage breakdown, especially if their spouses have a normal libido. These women need help.

Of course, we must look at all the other factors mentioned above, such as chronic health problems, drug use, alcohol, depression, and so on. Unfortunately, one of the main factors in women is often a relationship problem.

No hormones or herbs or nutrients or medicines can help this. Marriage/relationship counselling is needed, or a divorce lawyer!

I remember the answer one gynaecologist gave years ago when asked how he would treat poor libido in a woman. He said, tongue in cheek, *"get a new boyfriend!"*

As with men, women may also have a low libido with their husbands, but not with their boyfriends!

Relationship is a very important factor.

Once all these have been assessed and dealt with,

and there is still a low to nil libido, then hormones can be considered.

Testosterone has been described as the hormone of desire. Testosterone can be supplemented to women, although not on its own: it should be a part of general hormonal replacement, preferably natural/bioidentical.

Lobo, Rosen, Yang, Block, and Van Der Hoop (2003) showed that supplementing women with oestrogen and testosterone can significantly improve sexual functioning. Note that this study used synthetic hormones: esterified oestrogen and methyltestosterone.

Supplementing testosterone alone to women with *"Hypoactive Sexual Desire Disorder"* can improve libido (Davis et al., 2008).

Women seem to do well with oestrogen and testosterone replacement. However, in practice, I have found progesterone and testosterone a much better combination. In fact, I rarely prescribe oestrogen and testosterone only.

Anecdotally, I have found that progesterone alone can improve libido.

This is confirmed by Spark, Dunn, and Houlahan (2009) who surveyed women on their experience with compounded progesterone cream. *"Participating* *women gained symptom relief for migraine, painful breasts, mood swings, bloating, hot flushes, and other conditions. The participants also experienced unexpected benefits such as improvement in irregular and painful periods, relief from cystitis, or <u>increased libido</u>, without any reported negative side effects."* (Emphasis the author.)

Roney and Simmons (2013) showed that progesterone was a negative predictor of libido. On the other hand, Pillsworth, Haselton, and Buss (2004) showed an increase in libido in women in a long-term stable relationship compared to single women. The researchers state that *"Women's reproductive biology imposes heavy obligatory costs of parental investment, creating strong selective forces hypothesized to shape female mating psychology around critical decisions such as the choice of partner, the timing of sexual intercourse, and the timing of reproduction."*

This suggests that libido is not just related to hormones.

Then why does prescribing progesterone cream in women increase libido?

There may be a few reasons.

1) Low libido can be due to a relative excess of oestrogen (oestrogen dominance). We live in a polluted

world. Many of the pollutants are oestrogenic (xenoestrogens). Progesterone supplementation may balance out the excess effects of the xenoestrogens. Balance is the keyword.

2) Progesterone can be converted to testosterone.

3) Progesterone is made by the *corpus luteum,* which is formed after ovulation. Here, we can speculate that from a purely biological perspective, if the woman has ovulated, progesterone levels rise and an increase in libido will increase the chance of fertilisation.

There is one particular condition where I would consider it mandatory to replace not just oestrogen and progesterone but testosterone as well. This special condition is in women who have had a hysterectomy with bilateral oophorectomy.

Hysterectomy is a surgical procedure to remove the uterus. A "total hysterectomy" involves the removal of the uterus as well as both ovaries (bilateral oophorectomy). This procedure is very common; in 1993, a study in South Australia showed that at least one third of women would have a hysterectomy in their lifetime (MacLennan, MacLennan, & Wilson,1993).

However, hysterectomy rates decreased in Australia by 20% between 2014-15 to 2021-22. This is because of the increase in endometrial ablation. In a similar time frame, endometrial ablation increased by 10% between 2013-16 to 2019-22.

(https://www.safetyandquality.gov.au/our-work/healthcare-variation/womens-health-focus-report - accessed 7 July 2024)

Endometrial ablation is a surgical procedure where the inner lining of the uterus is removed/destroyed and this reduces and/or stops any bleeding. This technique is less invasive than hysterectomy, less traumatic, safer, and there is a much quicker recovery. It also achieves much the same result as a hysterectomy.

Why is this surgery done? In many cases, the surgery is done for symptoms of hormonal imbalance, such as fibroids and heavy bleeding. Other than the use of synthetic hormones, the only other treatment mainstream medicine knows is to "cut it out," although endometrial ablation is now becoming more popular.

This is not to say that there are some legitimate reasons for hysterectomy, and the principle one being cancer; but then, even uterine cancer and possibly cervical cancer may be hormonally caused. Be that as it may, women who have had hysterectomy, plus or minus oophorectomy (removal of ovaries), do not do so well.

"Hysterectomy has the potential for generating serious consequences in terms of health, including a two

to seven times greater incidence and prevalence of cardiovascular disease, and quality of life, including loss of sexual libido and pleasure" (Rako, 2000).

The ovaries are a critical source of oestrogen and make approximately half of circulating testosterone. Obviously, if the ovaries are removed, then this source is totally lost. Even in situations where the ovaries are spared, their function is compromised by removal of the uterus, as many of the arteries and veins are cut. Many of these women are put on oestrogen alone. Progesterone is not considered necessary, because there is no uterus. However, as we have seen earlier, this is not a valid reason because there are progesterone receptors all over the body.

In addition, many women suffer from a testosterone deficiency and are not treated because it is not recognised. Women who have had a hysterectomy with oophorectomy have a greater than 40% reduction in testosterone compared to women without surgery. Women with just hysterectomy showed intermediate levels (Laughlin, Barrett-Connor, Kritz-Silverstein, & von Mühlen, 2000).

Even in postmenopausal women, the ovary is still a critical source of testosterone. Testosterone replacement in these women not only improves quality of life in terms of libido and a sense of well-being, but also contributes to the prevention of osteoporosis and protection from cardiovascular disease.

In a study, 75 women aged 31-56 years who had hysterectomy with bilateral oophorectomy were treated with CEE and as well, randomly given either placebo, low dose testosterone patch or higher dose testosterone patch. The researchers concluded that *"In women who have undergone oophorectomy and hysterectomy, transdermal testosterone improves sexual function and psychological well-being"* (Shifren et al., 2000).

Sex hormone binding globulin (SHBG)

One important point I have not mentioned yet is that the sex hormones, notably oestrogens and testosterone, do *not* float freely in the blood. Ninety-eight percent of these hormones are bound to carrier proteins. Approximately 44% is bound to a glycoprotein called sex hormone binding globulin (SHBG), which is synthesized by the liver and approximately 54% is bound to albumin. Only about 2% is "free" and is therefore biologically active.

Note that SHBG has a greater affinity to bind to testosterone than to oestrogen.

The role of SHBG is to act as a storage, so that the hormone can be released as needed. The binding of the hormone to SHBG is quite strong, while the binding to albumin is weaker. This produces a tiered situation where the free hormone is obviously free, but the body can call on the albumin bound hormone at short notice. The hormone bound to the SHBG is more firmly bound and is more difficult to release and therefore use.

Testosterone physiology

Testosterone levels are monitored in the hypothalamus. Gonadotropin-releasing hormone (GnRH) is released from the hypothalamus and goes to the anterior pituitary gland via blood vessels, where it stimulates the release of luteinizing hormone (LH) which is secreted into the bloodstream. The LH travels to the Leydig cells in the testes, where it stimulates the production of testosterone. The blood level of testosterone forms a negative feedback loop to the hypothalamus, however, only the "free" testosterone and possibly the albumin bound testosterone can feedback to the hypothalamus.

In males, 95% of the testosterone is produced in the testes and only 5% comes from the adrenal glands.

GnRH stimulates the production and release of LH and follicle-stimulating hormone (FSH). In males, the GnRH is released in pulses at a regular frequency, while in women, the frequency of pulses varies during the menstrual cycle with a surge of GnRH just before ovulation.

In men, FSH stimulates the testes to produce sperm.

In women, approximately half of the testosterone

is made by the ovaries and half by the adrenal glands. The adrenal production of testosterone in women is not under the control of LH or FSH.

The ovaries make testosterone, but most is converted to oestrogen by the enzyme *aromatase*. Some testosterone is spared, which adds to the testosterone from the adrenal glands to exert its effects on female physiology. However, if the conversion to oestrogen is blocked, testosterone levels rise, which can cause many problems.

In women, FSH, assisted by LH, acts on the follicle to produce testosterone, which is then converted to oestrogen. LH stimulates ovulation.

In women, as well as men, there is a negative feedback loop to the hypothalamus, which regulates hormone levels. Hyperinsulinaemia increases the pulse activity of GnRH, leading to disordered LH and FSH activity as seen in polycystic ovarian syndrome (PCOS).

Knowing just the total testosterone level is not so helpful because we must know the level of SHBG and albumin. The bioavailability of the hormone is determined by the level of SHBG and albumin.

Scenario 1: Suppose total testosterone is low.

However, if SHBG is also low, then the "free" testosterone may be normal.

Scenario 2: Suppose total testosterone is normal. However, SHBG may be high and, therefore, the "free" testosterone can be low.

There can be many scenarios in-between!

There are two ways to regulate the level of "free" testosterone:

1) by increasing the total level of testosterone, and

2) by reducing the level of SHBG.

> The higher the SHBG, the lower the level of "free" testosterone.

In any assessment of hormone status, total testosterone, SHBG, albumin, and "free" testosterone need to be measured.

To deal with a hormone deficiency, we can look at ways to increase hormone levels, whether it be replacement, or herbs or nutrients. However, there is another way—we can influence the levels of SHBG. Since the whole system is quite dynamic, lowering SHBG will increase the "free" testosterone, although this may only be temporary. Too much "free" testosterone could negatively feed back to the hypothalamus and, overall, reduce LH, which will reduce testosterone secretion. Altering SHBG will only produce micro-variations of "free" testosterone in younger males, but may not be as significant in the elderly as the ageing testes are not as responsive to the LH. The levels of SHBG can be controlled by a balance of stimulating and inhibiting factors.

Below are two tables showing factors that can increase or decrease SHBG. You must remember that the body is a dynamic system, so these factors are never static.

Another important fact is that testosterone binds to SHBG much more strongly than to oestrogen, so if there is competition between oestrogen and testosterone for binding sites, testosterone wins. When more testosterone is bound, more oestrogen is "free". This may not be a good thing.

Table 1

Factors that increase SHBG

Age

Excess alcohol

Smoking

Hyperthyroidism, thyroid hormone, T3

Oestrogen, including phytoestrogen.

Low protein diet

High fibre diet

Table 2

Factors that decrease SHBG

Androgens

Progesterone

Cortisol

Hyperinsulinaemia, insulin, IGF-1

Obesity

Hypothyroidism

Hyperprolactinaemia

High protein, fat diet

Of course, addressing some of these factors can influence overall hormone levels.

One of the main factors that increases SHBG is ageing itself. As the male ages, SHBG goes up, and as well, the ageing testes make less testosterone, so the combination of a higher SHBG, which will bind more of the already depleted testosterone, will reduce the "free" testosterone level even more. This low "free" testosterone may stimulate the release of more LH, but the ageing testes may not be able to respond as readily.

Another factor associated with ageing is the increase in body fat and the decrease in muscle mass. These are related to low testosterone.

"...ageing in males is accompanied by an important increase in fat mass and a decrease in lean body mass. Several indices of body composition are significantly correlated with plasma testosterone levels before and after correction for BMI and age" (Vermeulen, Goemaere, & Kaufman,1999).

As mentioned above, body fat contains an enzyme called *aromatase,* which converts testosterone to oestrogen. So here we have a situation where the ageing male has more SHBG due to ageing as well as lower testosterone and more body fat, so that whatever testosterone he does have will be converted to oestrogen, which can in turn increase the SHBG.

This does not necessarily only happen in the ageing male: a younger, but obese male, can have similar problems. An obese male has more oestrogen that a non-obese male. This can readily be seen by the "man boobs"/ "moobs" on many obese males, young or old.

Let's take one step back. What causes a male (or even a female) to become obese?

One factor is the diet. The major cause of obesity in the western world is the refined carbohydrate and high-sugar diet. This diet consists of foods such as breads, pastries, cereals, sugar-laden soft drinks, refined pastas, noodles, and so on. All of which were never a part of the human diet until very recently. This highly refined carbohydrate diet induces hyperinsulinaemia, which, as we see in table 2, reduces the SHBG. This should be a good thing, as the lower SHBG would increase the free testosterone. Don't forget, however, that the negative feedback loop can reduce testosterone secretion.

Yes, but hyperinsulinaemia also encourages obesity so that the increased "free" testosterone is converted to oestrogen.

Hyperinsulinaemia in females can lead to polycystic ovarian syndrome (PCOS) where the women have high testosterone levels, are more hirsute, infertile and have multiple gynaecological issues, including polycystic ovaries.

There is some controversy about whether it is the hyperinsulinaemia or the sugar itself that reduces the SHBG. Perhaps it is both, or perhaps it is insulin resistance? Regardless, they are all related.

An early study showed an inverse relationship between insulin and SHBG. As insulin goes up, SHBG goes down; *"insulin controls SHBG synthesis in vivo"* (Strain, Zumoff, Rosner, & Pi-Sunyer, 1994).

This is where we get into a bind. If insulin goes up and SHBG goes down, doesn't that mean a high-sugar diet can reduce SHBG and produce more "free" testosterone? Isn't that a good thing, especially in older men? Certainly, however, in women, a higher testosterone may not be good!

In the context of this discussion, it is important to remember the negative feedback loop we discussed earlier that will reduce testosterone production.

We all know that a high-sugar diet can lead to hyperinsulinaemia and insulin resistance, which is not good; it produces many other problems.

How, then, if at all, does the onset of insulin resistance influence SHBG? During transition from pre-menopause to post-menopause, SHBG levels are increased in insulin sensitive women but decreased in insulin resistant women. In the pre-menopausal woman, the effect of oestradiol has a stronger action on SHBG levels than in the post-menopausal woman. In the post-menopausal woman, the impact of IR on SHBG is more important than the effect of oestradiol (Akin, Bastemir, & Alkis, 2007).

We know that in normal, healthy men, there is an inverse correlation between testosterone levels and insulin levels. As insulin levels rise, testosterone levels fall.

We also know that men with glucose intolerance and with type 2 diabetes (T2D) have lower testosterone levels than normal men do. There is an inverse correlation between IR and SHBG levels. This means that as IR increases, SHBG decreases. Insulin, therefore, is an important regulator of SHBG.

Some studies show an inverse relationship between testosterone levels and visceral fat mass, while other studies show low "free" testosterone in proportion to obesity. Testosterone is an important regulator of insulin sensitivity in men (Kapoor, Malkin, Channer, & Jones, 2005).

Why do obese men have lower testosterone? One suggestion is the hyperoestrogenaemia (too much oestrogen in blood).

The enzyme *aromatase* converts testosterone to oestrogen. This enzyme is in fat cells; therefore, the more fat cells present, the more *aromatase,* the more testosterone is converted to oestrogen. This leads to more oestrogen and less testosterone.

Another reason is that obesity is secondary to IR, which influences the Leydig cells in the testes, therefore, less testosterone is made (Pitteloud et al., 2005).

Furthermore, as insulin goes up, SHBG goes down, thus producing more "free" testosterone. This increased "free" testosterone activates the negative feedback loop to the hypothalamus, reducing the LH and therefore reducing testosterone production. So overall testosterone goes down as SHBG goes down.

I'm sorry if all this sounds too complicated … but it is!

If you read through again what we have already discussed, you can see that essentially diet influences insulin, which eventually results in IR, which can impact not just SHBG but testosterone production.

The underlying problem is insulin and IR. Obesity, one complication of IR, plays a major role.

Insulin and IR can influence hormones and SHBG.

Sugar itself can cause similar problems. Selva, Hogeveen, Innis, and Hammond (2007) showed that monosaccharides, such as glucose and fructose, reduced the production of SHBG in transgenic mice, as well as in human tissue cultures. The monosaccharides were converted to lipids, and this lipogenesis reduced the liver's ability to make the SHBG.

Sugar is very high in the western diet. Table sugar is a di-saccharide consisting of fructose and glucose. The most common sweetener in the USA is high fructose corn syrup (HFCS), which, as its name suggests, is high in fructose.

As SHBG is reduced, there is more "free" testosterone, which is not good for females. Initially, in men, there may be an increased level of "free" testosterone, however, testosterone levels reduce because of a feedback adjustment of gonadotropin secretion.

So, the high-sugar diet induces obesity, and the increased amount of *aromatase* converts some of that little amount of testosterone to oestrogen.

A high protein diet can also reduce SHBG. However, a high protein diet does not produce hyperinsulinaemia and obesity to the same extent as sugars. Therefore, a higher protein, lower sugar diet, will produce a reduced fat mass, which would mean a lower level of *aromatase.* The end result is that the higher level of "free" testosterone is not converted to oestrogen.

"We conclude that age and body mass index are
173

major determinants of SHBG concentration in older men, and fibre and protein intake are also significant contributors to SHBG levels, but total caloric intake and the intake of carbohydrate and fat are not significant. Thus, diets low in protein in elderly men may lead to elevated SHBG levels and decreased testosterone bioactivity. The decrease in bioavailable testosterone can then result in declines in sexual function and muscle and red cell mass, and contribute to the loss of bone density" (Longcope, Feldman, McKinlay, & Araujo, 2000).

It is interesting to note that in this study, carbohydrate intake did not seem to have an effect. However, in the Selva, Hogeveen, Innis, and Hammond (2007) study, high sugar did have an effect.

Diet and exercise can have a great impact on SHBG levels, which in turn can influence "free" testosterone.

Many studies have looked at the potential for diets to lower testosterone levels, mainly because of the idea that a high testosterone level can cause prostate cancer. In the situation of the ageing male, where testosterone levels are low, shouldn't we try to optimise testosterone levels instead of reducing them?

The dogma seems to be that testosterone causes

prostate cancer and, as we have seen, this is not strictly correct. Again, I will ask, if it is the testosterone alone, why does prostate cancer occur in the elderly where testosterone levels are on the decline? Prostate cancer is dependent on both oestrogen and testosterone; neither on its own is sufficient to evoke malignant growth (Risbridger, Bianco, Ellem, & McPherson, 2003).

There are probably other factors that are implicated in prostate cancer, including lifestyle, xenoestrogens, carcinogens, vitamin D deficiency, and zinc deficiency, to name a few.

Testosterone alone is not the problem. The elderly need to keep their testosterone levels up and their oestrogen levels down for reasons already mentioned.

Insulin, SHBG, prostate-specific antigen (PSA) and lipids were measured in obese men put on a *low fat, high fibre* diet plus exercise. Insulin decreased, SHBG increased, BMI decreased, and PSA levels remained the same except in a small sub-group of men who initially had elevated PSA levels, where the levels reduced. A low fat and exercise regime reduced androgen levels (Tymchuk, Tessler, Aronson, & Barnard,1998).

The purpose of the above study was to lower testosterone, which they considered a good thing. They showed diet can lower testosterone levels to "protect" against prostate cancer, which may not necessarily be correct.

Elderly men need to keep their testosterone levels up, or as near to normal as possible. One result of this study, however, was beneficial. The lowering of insulin levels is definitely a good thing. The lowering of PSA in a small sub-group could also have been due to the lowered insulin.

Omnivorous men were compared with vegetarian men. The researchers found that there was a higher level of SHBG and a lower level of free androgen index (FAI) among the vegetarians.

"The increases in androstane-3 alpha, 17 beta-diol glucuronide and androstane-3 beta, 17 beta-diol glucuronide levels in the omnivorous group are probably a consequence of the elevation of the FAI. Our data suggest that in a vegetarian group, less testosterone is available for androgenic action" (Bélanger et al., 1989).

I should point out that what is more important is the level of SHBG that controls the level of "free" testosterone rather than the effect it has on total testosterone.

In another study, the researchers look at the post-prandial (after meal) effect of different meals on serum testosterone. As men are post-prandial for a significant portion of the day, this effect is important. A significant decrease in testosterone and free androgen index (FAI) was found after both a tofu meal and a lean meat meal. Here again, the researchers suggested this to be a good thing, that is, a low-fat diet to reduce testosterone levels (Habito & Ball, 2001).

The above studies considered keeping testosterone low to be a good thing. I disagree. Testosterone levels need to be kept up.

So, to raise testosterone, we should do the opposite to what the researchers suggest, that is, eat a diet higher in fat and protein and low in sugar. Therefore, to raise testosterone, one shouldn't be eating tofu or a diet low in animal fat.

Testosterone and exercise

As we have seen, ageing is associated with a decline in physiological function which can be related to a decrease in growth hormone (GH) levels and testosterone levels. Some previous studies used exercise, in conjunction with diet to influence testosterone levels. Exercise is important. Ageing males tend to be less active, but is this a chicken or the egg scenario?

Is it the lower testosterone due to ageing that causes the lower activity levels, or are lower activity levels the cause of the lower testosterone?

Possibly it is the latter. Hurel et al. (1999) looked at exercise in runners and noted that *"...results suggest that regular intensive exercise in older male subjects is associated with higher growth hormone and testosterone levels and that exercise may have a role in countering the normal decline in growth hormone with ageing."*

Exercise seems to produce a higher level of testosterone in men and women, which would be advantageous for a better sex life. However, a good sex life is dependent on a fitter and healthier body.

Bortz and Wallace (1999) concluded that *"... sexual satisfaction seemed to correlate with the degree of fitness. We conclude that physical fitness and high levels of sexual activity are mutually supportive elements of successful ageing."*

However, one must be careful.

Is it the exercise?

or

Is it that men with higher testosterone can do the exercise?

Men with lower testosterone are too tired, weak, or not motivated enough to do exercise. Therefore, looking at men who exercise, may give a biased picture.

The same with sex.

Davey Smith, Frankel, and Yarnell (1997) showed that men who have more sex/more orgasms per week live longer.

Is it that sex produces longevity, or is it that healthier men can have more sex?

Billups, Bank, Padma-Nathan, Katz, and Williams (2005) showed that ED can be viewed as an early indicator of systemic cardiovascular disease.

Men with ED have damaged arteries and are therefore more prone to heart disease and are, obviously, less likely to be able to have sex.

Men without ED have better arteries, are less likely to die of heart disease, and therefore, are more likely to have sex.

The chicken or the egg scenario again!

Hall, Shackelton, Rosen, and Araujo (2010) clarified this to some extent. Sex is good for men. Their study showed that it is the *reduced* level of sexual activity that is associated with higher death rate due to heart disease *independent* of ED. So, *not* having sex is bad for men's health.

Sexual interest and activity in itself can increase testosterone levels (Stoléru, Ennaji, Cournot, & Spira, 1993).

This can apply to women as well. Exercise in women can also increase testosterone, which can be considered the hormone of libido. Women generally feel more sexual after an exercise workout. Sex can increase levels of testosterone.

van Anders, Hamilton, Schmidt, and Watson (2007) showed that even cuddling can increase testosterone levels in women.

In some ways, a close physical relationship becomes a self-perpetuating mechanism. Close physical contact can increase testosterone which can increase libido and produce more physical contact.

Sex can also be considered as exercise!

Back to exercise, although don't forget that sex can

be considered as a form of exercise!

"With training the older group demonstrated a significant increase in total testosterone in response to exercise stress along with significant decreases in resting cortisol. These data indicate that older men do respond with an enhanced hormonal profile in the early phase of a resistance training program, but the response is different from that of younger men" (Kraemer et al., 1999).

So, you can see that there are complex interactions between ageing, diet, and exercise; in the end these factors, positive and negative balance out and determine a level of free androgen. This process is not a static state, rather it is fluid and changes continually.

Nevertheless, by making a good life and healthy choices, the levels can be optimised. Of course, ageing cannot be altered too much, but diet and exercise can. By reducing sugar and increasing fat and protein, SHBG levels and "free" testosterone can be maximised. Encouraging exercise in whatever form is also very important.

The bottom line is that many elderly men have poor diets, generally low in protein and higher in sugars, and exercise less than they did when younger.

So, to optimise hormonal health for elderly males,

they should be encouraged to:

1) exercise more,
2) have more sex,
3) be less stressed,
4) eat more protein, and
5) eat less sugar and refined carbohydrates.

"Feed the man meat!"

On the other hand, poor dietary choices can increase SHBG, which will reduce "free" testosterone. Younger males will compensate by increasing LH secretion, which will stimulate testosterone production but, in the elderly the feedback loop will not increase testosterone secretion due to the state of the ageing testes.

In women, nutritional factors are now recognised to be more important in SHBG regulation than sex steroid levels.

"Although sex steroids have long been known to influence serum concentrations of SHBG, it is now recognized that nutritional factors may be more important in the regulation of SHBG in women. Thus,

SHBG concentrations are negatively correlated with body mass index (BMI) and, more particularly, to indices of central adiposity. Polycystic ovary syndrome (PCOS), the most common cause of anovulatory infertility, is associated with truncal obesity, hyperandrogenism and hyperinsulinaemia. There is evidence that insulin may be the humoral mediator of the weight-dependent changes in SHBG. Serum SHBG concentrations are inversely correlated with both fasting and glucose-stimulated insulin levels, and insulin has been shown to have a direct inhibitory effect on SHBG synthesis and secretion by hepatocytes in culture. However, the interrelationship of BMI, insulin and SHBG appears to be different in women with PCOS from that in normal subjects. The clinical importance of the weight-related suppression of SHBG is illustrated by the finding of a greater prevalence of hirsutism in obese women PCOS compared with their lean counterparts. Obese subjects with PCOS have similar total testosterone concentrations to lean PCO women but have lower SHBG and reciprocally higher free testosterone levels. Calorie restriction results in reduction of serum insulin followed by an increase in SHBG and a fall in free testosterone but an isocaloric, low-fat diet has no significant effect on SHBG concentrations. Weight reduction in obese, hyperandrogenaemic women with PCOS is an important approach to the management of both anovulation and

183

hirsutism" (Botwood, Hamilton-Fairley, Kiddy, Robinson, & Franks,1995).

Aromatase

Aromatase is the enzyme responsible for the conversion of testosterone to oestrogens. The enzyme is found in many tissues including gonads, brain, placenta, blood vessels, skin, bone, and endometrium, although it is mainly found in fat cells in both sexes. Obviously, the action of this enzyme must be different in women and men. Men want to reduce the effect of *aromatase* and hang onto their testosterone. Women want to convert most of their testosterone to oestrogen. There is a gender difference in the regulation of a*romatase* (McTernan et al., 2000; McTernan et al., 2002).

Insulin, in the presence of follicle-stimulating hormone (FSH) is known to stimulate *aromatase* activity. So, how does this tie in with the observed fact that in the condition known as PCOS, testosterone is elevated, and oestrogen is low.

PCOS has been linked with MetS, which has as its underlying basis an elevated insulin level (hyperinsulinaemia), and a resultant insulin resistance.

But shouldn't the high insulin levels continue to

stimulate *aromatase?* Insulin *does* increase *aromatase* activity, but only up to a point. Insulin at concentrations of 0.5, 1 and 10 ng/ml stimulates activity. However, at higher insulin doses (100ng/ml), *aromatase* is not activated (Bhatia & Price, 2001).

When there is hyperinsulinaemia, which is found in PCOS, the high insulin suppresses *aromatase.* The hypothalamus, sensing a low oestrogen secretes FSH which stimulates the ovaries to make testosterone but cannot convert it to oestrogen. The hypothalamus still sensing a low oestrogen releases more FSH, and the cycle continues. Testosterone levels increase which has a deleterious effect on the female body.

The main thrust of treatment of PCOS is to reduce insulin levels and to improve the insulin resistance. Other than conversion to oestrogen by *aromatase,* testosterone can also be converted to di hydro testosterone (DHT) by the enzyme *5-alpha reductase.*

Di-hydro testosterone (DHT)

DHT is the biologically active metabolite of testosterone and is a much more potent androgen. The main sites of production are in the prostate, testes, hair follicles and adrenal glands. Testosterone is converted to

DHT by the enzyme *5-alpha reductase*. DHT is three times more potent than testosterone and is best known for its role in producing male pattern baldness and prostate problems.

The role of DHT is mainly during embryonic life where the hormone is responsible for the development of primary male sex characteristics. It is also crucial during puberty for the development of the male sex-specific characteristics, such as facial and body hair, deepening of the voice, sex drive and growth of muscles.

In later life, DHT continues to have a very important role in male sexual function.

One important fact about DHT is that it cannot be aromatised, i.e. a*romatase* cannot convert it to oestrogen.

DHT cannot be aromatised.

Testosterone and DHT have long been accused of being the main factors in the development of prostate cancer and benign prostatic hypertrophy (BPH). For a long time, the dogma was *not* to give testosterone or DHT because these androgens would "feed" the prostate cancer and encourage growth. For many years this idea seemed set in concrete, however, lately, the idea is changing. Newer studies have shown that testosterone and/or DHT are not solely responsible for BPH or prostate cancer.

Marks et al. (2006) studied hypogonadal men who were given either testosterone injections or a placebo injection. The researchers also did prostate biopsies at baseline and after six months. Blood tests showed that serum testosterone levels rose with testosterone replacement, however when the tissue from the prostate biopsy was analysed in the testosterone group, there was no increase in testosterone or DHT in the prostatic tissue.

Another study looked at DHT levels in serum and from prostate tissue in men with different Gleeson scores. Gleeson score is a grading system (2-10) devised by Dr Donald Gleeson in 1977, for prostate cancer. Low scores are less aggressive and less likely to spread. High scores are very aggressive and are more likely to spread. DHT was shown to be *lower* in the high Gleeson scores, i.e. in the more aggressive tumours (Nishiyama, Ikarashi, Hashimoto, Suzuki, & Takahashi, 2006).

So, if androgens need to be supplemented, why isn't DHT supplemented, instead of testosterone?

That is a fair question to ask.

In an animal experiment, prostate-cancer susceptible male rats were given either DHT or testosterone injections. After 14 months, prostate adenocarcinoma developed in 24% of the testosterone treated rats but none developed in the DHT treated rats (Pollard, Snyder, & Luckert, 1987).

Does this rat experiment have any relevance to humans?

Possibly.

Since DHT is *not* aromatised, this would make it attractive to use in androgen therapy instead of testosterone.

"A 1.8 years survey of 37 men aged 55-70 years treated with daily percutaneous DHT treatment suggested that high plasma levels of DHT (>8.5 nmol/l) effectively induced clinical benefits while slightly but significantly reducing prostate size" (de Lignieres, 1993).

This study concluded that DHT could even shrink an enlarged prostate.

Kunelius, Linukkarinen, Hannuksela, Itkonen, and Tapanainen (2002) also used transdermal DHT for six months in 120 ageing males. Investigations showed no adverse effects. Prostate weight and PSA levels did not change.

So, DHT is not as dangerous as originally thought. In fact, DHT probably is more beneficial than testosterone.

Why?

Although prostate cancer and BPH need androgens such as testosterone and DHT to develop, they act in more of a permissive role, that is, on their own, the androgens are insufficient to cause these problems. There is a missing factor, and that missing factor is oestrogen.

Both androgens and oestrogens are needed to produce the problem.

When testosterone is supplemented, aromatisation can convert some of the testosterone to oestrogen, and then you have both testosterone and oestrogen to cause problems.

When supplementing testosterone, an *aromatase* inhibitor would be highly recommended. One *aromatase* inhibitor is zinc, a mineral that is generally deficient in western societies (Om & Chung, 1996).

Supplementing DHT will not produce oestrogen and is, therefore, much safer.

189

BPH is found in men who have an increased ratio of oestrogen to androgen levels, i.e. higher oestrogen, lower testosterone (Wynder, Nicholson, DeFranco, & Ricke, 2015).

So, why does the use of a *5-alpha reductase* inhibitor reduce the size of the prostate? Remember, *5-alpha reductase* is the enzyme that converts testosterone to DHT.

The simplistic view of BPH is that the testosterone is converted to DHT by the enzyme *5-alpha reductase* and this more potent androgen stimulates the prostate to grow and therefore cause the BPH. The simplistic way to deal with this is to give a drug that blocks the *5-alpha reductase*. There are drugs on the market that have this action, although the results are not that good. They claim that the drugs reduce the prostate size by 30%. This is a reasonable reduction, but if it is only the DHT that is involved, then the results *should* be better.

We know that testosterone levels decline as we age. How could a hormone that is declining be the cause of the problem?

We have also seen that SHBG increases with age, which also reduces the level of "free" testosterone even more.

So, I ask again, how could a declining level of

testosterone be a cause for BPH, or cancer for that matter?

Unless a *lack* of testosterone is a cause.

There must be another mechanism.

Prostate enlargement is not reliant on testosterone levels but on the ratio of oestrogen to testosterone. Yes, oestrogen, the "female" hormone. With ageing, the level of oestrogen goes up, while the level of testosterone goes down. In the prostate, DHT levels remain stable, but oestrogen levels go up.

There is a second hormonal pathway where oestrogens can mimic androgens.

Here, the surprising fact is that SHBG itself acts as a hormone. Nakhla, Romas, and Rosner (1997) showed that SHBG attaches to a specific sex hormone binding globulin receptor (RSHBG). This SHBG-RSHBG complex is activated by oestradiol and stimulates the receptor to increase growth factors, which in turn causes the prostate to grow.

Here we have a situation where there is low testosterone, high oestrogen, and high SHBG; this combination has an androgenic-like growth action on the prostate (Farnsworth, 1996).

To treat BPH, firstly the oestrogen levels need to be kept low. This can be done by inhibiting *aromatase*. Zinc is a very useful mineral in that it not only acts as an *aromatase* inhibitor but also can act as a *5-alpha reductase* inhibitor. Low levels of zinc can increase activity while higher doses can inhibit activity (Leake, Chisholm, & Habib, 1984).

Another *aromatase* inhibitor is chrysin which will be discussed later.

SHBG also needs to be kept low, and this was discussed earlier.

Testosterone levels need to be elevated, and this has also been discussed.

Herbs can also be used in this situation, and these will be discussed later.

Dehydroepiandrosterone (DHEA)

Dehydroepiandrosterone (DHEA) is a steroid hormone produced by the adrenal gland and is perhaps the most abundant steroid found in humans. Over 90% of the DHEA is converted to DHEA-sulphate (DHEA-s) and from here it can be re-converted back to DHEA or to other hormones such as oestrogen, testosterone, progesterone, cortisol, and others. This is why it has been described as the "mother hormone." However, it cannot simply be regarded as a reservoir hormone (i.e. acts as a form of storage to make other hormones as necessary); it has its own spectrum of action although this is vaguely understood.

So not only is DHEA a buffer and a "mother hormone", but it can also be considered a "pre-hormone" and a hormone stimulator.

In Australia, DHEA can only be obtained by prescription from a registered medical practitioner and dispensed from a compounding pharmacist. In the USA, DHEA is available over the counter in pharmacies and health food shops, although there are moves afoot to try to either ban it or to make it prescription only.

Do not get confused.

Some of my patients have told me that they have bought DHEA from the local health food shop. I suggest that you all look closely at what you are buying. These are homeopathic forms, generally in the 6x potency of DHEA. Note that 6x refers to a homeopathic potency, not that it is 6 times as potent.

This, of course, does not mean that they do not work. This also does not belittle homeopathy or homeopathic remedies. Some get great benefit from these products. The point I am trying to make is that if you want DHEA in physiological quantities, then it can only be obtained by prescription from a registered medical practitioner who has studied natural hormones.

DHEA is a very useful and versatile hormone.

It is similar to the other steroid hormones. It can act on androgenic receptors, although there are also specific DHEA receptors found on endothelial cells (Liu & Dillon, 2002).

The known actions of DHEA include,

- Regulates hormones through specific or non-specific hormone receptors.
- Inhibits an anti-proliferative enzyme, G-6-PD.
- Increases fat metabolism through thermogenesis.

- Decreases desire to eat, possibly through its effects on insulin.
- Decreases stress reaction.
- Stimulates T-lymphocytes.
- Enhances interleukin 2 production.
- Improves calcium absorption/anti-osteoporotic.
- Anti-inflammatory activity.

DHEA is found in high concentrations, equal to that of the adrenal cortex, in the brain and nervous system. Some brain cells, specifically the astrocytes, can manufacture DHEA (Zwain & Yen, 1999).

One important point to highlight is that most of this research was done on rat brains. What about human brains? We do know that DHEA is abundant in the human brain, but can human brains make DHEA? It seems that oligodendrocytes and astrocytes can produce DHEA, but neurons cannot (Brown, Cascio, & Papadopoulos, 2000).

Since the brain produces DHEA, we must conclude that DHEA has some purpose relating to brain function. However, we are not sure what that role is.

DHEA is perhaps the most abundant steroid hormone in the body, levels peak around the age of 21 and slowly decline with ageing. At its peak, men produce approximately 31 mg, and women, 19 mg daily. By age 75, levels have decreased by 80-90%. This decline has led to the thought that replacing DHEA could be like giving an "anti-ageing" hormone.

So, what is its function? We know a lot about what it can do but we truly do not know where, or how, it all fits into the scheme of things.

The great DHEA scam

For many years, DHEA was known as the "Fountain of Youth" hormone, mainly because levels peak at age 21 and slowly decline thereafter. These two were associated and the popular theory was that ageing is related to DHEA levels; therefore, to treat "ageing", DHEA could be supplemented. This led to much hype and for a while DHEA became a "wonder hormone" used for all aspects of ageing. Many benefits were attributed to DHEA, including anti-ageing, improved muscle mass, loss of weight, greater sexual performance, clearer thinking, and so on, although studies have shown conflicting results.

In the past, products were released onto the market claiming to be DHEA. On closer inspection, the product was not DHEA but wild yam (*Dioscorea villosa*) extract, with the claim that the body converts the wild yam extract into DHEA. The small print on the label called the product a "DHEA precursor". Wild yam cream is still being made but no longer with the "DHEA precursor" claim.

It is true that to manufacture DHEA, an extract from wild yam, *diosgenin*, can be converted to DHEA with a 5-6 step laboratory process. However, the human body does not have the machinery to achieve this.

About the same time, other products claiming to be progesterone were released. This also, on closer inspection, was a wild yam extract, a "progesterone precursor" claiming that the wild yam was converted into progesterone. This is a false claim as the body cannot convert diosgenin to progesterone.

Just a note here, some do respond very well to wild yam cream, but this is not because it is DHEA or progesterone, rather because it is a phytoestrogen.

Progesterone is manufactured from wild yam and this process is also done in the laboratory.

A little time later, "real" DHEA was released onto the USA market, again with great hype and fanfare. One group claimed DHEA to be the "wonder hormone". The mainstream claimed that DHEA was worthless. What is the truth?

Like all other things in medicine, the truth is somewhere in- between.

DHEA: What can it do?

DHEA does have benefits - when given in the right amount, in the correct context, to the appropriate people, by doctors who are experienced in its use.

Some studies show no benefits of DHEA replacement (Flynn, Weaver-Osterholtz, Sharpe-Timms, Allen, & Krause, 1999; Arle et al., 2001; Nair et al., 2006) while others do show benefit.

We know that abnormal patterns of DHEA are associated with several disease states and dysfunction. These include chronic depression, chronic infections, chronic fatigue syndrome, osteoporosis, AIDS, hypoglycaemia, hypo and hyper adrenal function, stress response, many types of cancer, obesity, hypothyroidism, and Alzheimer's disease. Here again we genuinely do not know if it is the chicken or the egg!

The fact that, with some disease states, low DHEA levels have been found, led to trials of DHEA being supplemented, with varying results.

The mainstream view is that DHEA replacement has no place in medical practice. However, as we shall see in the following abstracts, DHEA has been shown to have positive effects.

In their study of metabolic effects of DHEA replacement in postmenopausal women, Lasco et al. (2000) found that *"Long-term treatment with DHEA ameliorates some metabolic parameters that are linked to increased cardiovascular risk and, consequently, this seems to be an interesting therapeutic tool in the management of the postmenopausal syndrome."*

While in their study of the effects of DHEA replacement in men and women of advancing age, Morales, Nolan, Nelson, and Yen (1994) concluded that *"... restoring DHEA and DS (DHEA-s) to young adult levels in men and women of advancing age induced an increase in the bioavailability of IGF-I, as reflected by an increase in IGF-I and a decrease in IGFBP-1 levels. These observations together with improvement of physical and psychological well-being in both genders and the absence of side-effects constitute the first demonstration of novel effects of DHEA replacement in age-advanced men and women*

199

Bloch, Schmidt, Danaceau, Adams, and Rubinow (1999) studied DHEA treatment of midlife dysthymia and noted that *"This pilot study suggests that dehydroepiandrosterone is an effective treatment for midlife-onset dysthymia."*

Dysthymia is a milder, but long-lasting form of depression, and the word is also used to describe a *"bad state of mind"* or *"ill humour."*

DHEA monotherapy in midlife-onset major and minor depression was found by Schmidt et al. (2005) *"… to be an effective treatment for midlife-onset major and minor depression."*

In the context of the DHEAge study, Baulieu et al. (2000) discussed what happened when *"Two hundred and eighty healthy individuals (women and men 60-79 years old) were given DHEA, 50 mg, or placebo, orally, daily for a year in a double-blind, placebo-controlled study."*

The researchers found that *"No potentially harmful accumulation of DHEAS and active steroids was recorded. Besides the reestablishment of a "young" concentration of DHEAS, a small increase of testosterone and estradiol was noted, particularly in women, and may be involved in the significantly demonstrated physiological-clinical manifestations here reported. Bone turnover improved selectively in women >70 years old, as assessed by the dual-energy x-ray absorptiometry (DEXA) technique and the decrease of osteoclastic activity. A significant increase in most libido parameters was also found in these older women. Improvement of the skin status was observed, particularly in women, in terms of hydration, epidermal thickness, sebum production, and pigmentation. A number of biological indices confirmed the lack of harmful consequences of this 50 mg/day DHEA administration over one year, also indicating that this kind of replacement therapy normalized some effects of aging, but does not create "supermen/women" (doping)."*

The effects of DHEA replacement on bone mineral density and body composition in elderly women and men were studied by Villareal, Holloszy, and Kohrt in 2000. The authors were optimistic about the outcome, stating that *"The results provide preliminary evidence that DHEA replacement in those elderly women and men who have very low serum DHEAS levels can partially reverse age-related changes in fat mass, fat-free mass, and BMD, and raise the possibility that increases in IGF-I and/or testosterone play a role in mediating these effects of DHEA."*

Villareal and Holloszy (2004) conducted a randomised controlled trial to see what effect DHEA had on abdominal fat and insulin action in elderly women and men. The authors cautiously stated that *"DHEA replacement could play a role in prevention and treatment of the metabolic syndrome associated with abdominal obesity."*

In a review of prospective and retrospective studies, the authors Thijs, Fagard, Forette, Nawrot, and Staessen (2003) were able to find conclusive evidence that low DHEA levels are predictive for cardiovascular diseases. *"The present findings suggest that, in men, low serum levels of DHEAS may be associated with coronary heart disease. However, whether DHEA supplementation has any cardiovascular benefit is not clear. Data from prospective randomised trials are needed."*

Kawano et al. (2003) found that DHEA supplementation improves endothelial function and insulin sensitivity in men. *"The low dose DHEA supplementation improves vascular endothelial function and insulin sensitivity and decreases the plasminogen activator inhibitor type 1 concentration. These beneficial changes have the potential to attenuate the development of age-related disorders such as cardiovascular disease."*

There is one situation where DHEA replacement can be very useful and that is in Addison's disease. Since the majority of DHEA is manufactured by the adrenal glands, it makes sense to replace this hormone if there is no adrenal function.

Long-term DHEA replacement in primary adrenal insufficiency was found to be helpful by Gurnell et al. (2008) who wrote that *"Although further long-term studies of DHEA therapy, with dosage adjustment, are desirable, our results support some beneficial effects of prolonged DHEA treatment in Addison's disease."*

A few years before the Gurnell study, Hunt et al. (2000) were encouraged by the results of their randomised double-blind trial. They found DHEA replacement improved mood and fatigue in those with Addison's disease who took part in the trial. *"Our results indicate that DHEA replacement corrects this steroid deficiency effectively and improves some aspects of psychological function. Beneficial effects in males, independent of circulating testosterone levels, suggest that it may act directly on the central nervous system rather than by augmenting peripheral androgen biosynthesis. These positive effects, in the absence of significant adverse events, suggest a role for DHEA replacement therapy in the treatment of Addison's disease."*

Dr Peter Baratosy MBBS FACNEM

DHEA and cancer

There is always the fear that hormones can cause cancer.

Does DHEA cause cancer? After all, DHEA can be converted to oestrogen, and oestrogen has been classed as a carcinogen. DHEA is also an androgenic hormone. Until recently, the fear was that testosterone could promote prostate cancer, however, as we have previously seen, newer research has shown that testosterone does not specifically cause prostate cancer.

What about DHEA?

For every study that shows DHEA causes cancer, there is a study which shows exactly the opposite.

It is important to be aware of the fact that many of these studies have been done, and new ones continue to be done, in animal models. And so, the question must be asked: *"What relationship is there between cancer in the animal model and humans?"*

Animal and test tube studies show that DHEA may reduce or prevent cancer. DHEA has been shown to have an anti-proliferative effect on malignant cell lines in experimental animals (Jiang et al., 2005).

204

DHEA is a glucose-6-phosphate dehydrogenase (G6PD) inhibitor and is considered one of the mechanisms that has chemo preventative and anti-proliferative actions on tumours.

"Epidemiological and experimental studies suggest that dehydroepiandrosterone (DHEA) exerts a protective effect against breast cancer. It has been proposed that the non-competitive inhibition of glucose-6-phosphate dehydrogenase (G6PD) contributes to DHEA antitumor action." "DHEA inhibition of G6PD was only found to occur at concentrations above 10 microM." The authors continued *"In contrast, at concentrations in the in vivo breast tissue concentration range, neither cell growth nor enzyme activity was inhibited. The results failed to confirm DHEA's putative anti-tumor action on breast cancer through G6PD inhibition, as the enzyme blockade only becomes apparent at pharmacological concentrations of the steroid"* (Di Monaco et al., 1997).

This is not the only mechanism as *"... results demonstrate that endogenous DHEA metabolites also have an anti-proliferative action that is not induced by inhibiting G6PD or HMGR activity alone"* (Yoshida et al., 2003).

Another problem is that many of the studies only look at DHEA. Cancer is a multi-factorial issue and

205

looking at only one variable is insufficient to get a true picture of the whole person. One of the studies quoted below, however, does look at obesity, which is known to be associated with breast cancer via hyperinsulinaemia and insulin resistance.

There is much confusion as is evident from the outcomes of the studies below.

*DHEA does not cause cancer in premenopausal women.

"Our analysis did not reveal a relationship between DHEA or DHEA-S and subsequent breast cancer in middle-aged premenopausal women" (Page et al., 2004).

*DHEA does cause cancer in premenopausal women.

"Our results suggest that adrenal androgens are positively associated with breast cancer among predominantly premenopausal women" (Tworoger et al., 2006).

*DHEA does not cause cancer in postmenopausal women.

"No evidence was found of an association between DHEAS and risk of breast cancer in postmenopausal

women." (Zeleniuch-Jacquotte et al., 1997).

*DHEA <u>does</u> cause cancer in postmenopausal women.

"Late promotion of breast cancer in postmenopausal women may be stimulated by prolonged intake of DHEA, and the risk may be increased by the endocrine abnormality associated with pre-existing abdominal obesity. Caution is advised in the use of dietary supplements of DHEA particularly by obese postmenopausal women" (Stoll, 1999).

Osawa et al. (2002) looked at colon cancer and showed that DHEA did reduce aberrant crypt foci (ACF). *"The number of ACF was significantly decreased in mice treated with 0.4% (p < 0.001) and 0.8% DHEA (p < 0.001), but there were no significant differences between DHEA-treated and control mice in terms of the ACF size, 3-catenin expression or level of dysplasia. This is the first study of colon cancer carcinogenesis demonstrating that DHEA treatment can decrease the number of ACF without apparently modifying their malignant potential. These data strongly suggest that DHEA might be a potential chemopreventative agent against human colon cancer."*

Note: this study was done on a mouse model.

Suh-Burgmann, Sivret, Duska, Del Carmen, and Seiden (2003) showed that intra-vaginal DHEA can improve early cervical cancer and dysplasia.

Aoki et al. (2003) concluded *"Thus, since DHEA has many beneficial effects experimentally, we should consider administration of DHEA in the future, and common mechanisms among these actions of DHEA should be elucidated in further studies."*

Is the notion that DHEA has a relationship to cancer so far-fetched? After all, cancer is more common in the elderly when DHEA level is low and progressively going southward!

Cancer does not generally occur in the young when DHEA levels are high. (This same argument can be used for testosterone and prostate cancer.)

Perhaps it is that low DHEA causes cancer. Perhaps supra-physiological replacement may cause cancer but what about physiological supplementation of DHEA?

With any supplementation it is important to replace only the amount needed to raise levels to normal, and not take huge, un-regulated doses, which may cause issues. I again stress that the levels need to be monitored.

Howard (2007) suggests that *low* levels of DHEA are the common factor of cancer and MetS.

Cortisol steal

A low DHEA is a de facto measurement of adrenal function. From the diagram you can see how this may occur.

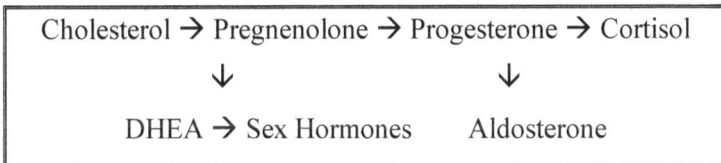

Cholesterol → Pregnenolone → Progesterone → Cortisol

↓ ↓

DHEA → Sex Hormones   Aldosterone

In order to make more cortisol to deal with the stress, the biochemical route goes more to cortisol production (the "cortisol highway") which therefore results in a reduced pathway to DHEA. This is referred to as "cortisol steal." Also, to make more cortisol, larger amounts of the starting raw ingredient, which just happens to be cholesterol, are needed. This is possibly why stress is another reason for elevated cholesterol levels.

Also, as the main pathway is to cortisol, less DHEA is made (as we have already seen) therefore fewer sex hormones are produced. These lower levels of sex hormones lead to hormone imbalance and menstrual irregularity in women and sexual difficulties in men associated with stress.

For the same reason, there is less going towards the making of aldosterone. Aldosterone is a hormone that controls kidney reabsorption of sodium and water. As there is less aldosterone, the salt and water are not reabsorbed by the kidneys and this leads to more frequent urination, salt loss and a subsequent salt craving, which are both signs of "adrenal fatigue". When you are stressed, you do tend to pee more!

This low DHEA, with possible associated high cortisol, or just overall hypofunction of the gland, can be related to overall low immune function. Could this reduction of immune surveillance be one reason for cancer development?

Could they be related at all?

In the end, what can we conclude?

DHEA probably does not cause cancer. DHEA deficiency could be related to cancer development due to stress causing a disordered adrenal function.

Endogenous Hormones and Prostate Cancer Collaborative Group; Roddam, Allen, Appleby, and Key (2008) performed an analysis of the existing worldwide epidemiological data to examine if there is any association between endogenous sex hormones (which includes DHEA) and prostate cancer.

They concluded that *"In this collaborative analysis of the worldwide data on endogenous hormones and prostate cancer risk, serum concentrations of sex hormones were not associated with the risk of prostate cancer."*

What can be plainer than that?

DHEA or any other androgenic hormone does not cause prostate cancer.

DHEA replacement must be:

1) individually based,
2) replaced physiologically to "youthful levels,"
3) monitored regularly.

Römmler (2003) wrote, *"We suggest replacement therapy in cases of adrenopause with an "individually adjusted" low DHEA dose between 5 and 50 mg for women and 15 and 100 mg for men in order to raise DS peak levels into the physiological range of younger adults. This procedure has here been applied routinely for the last 5 years, leading to an excellent compliance of the patients. In contrast, a high-dose pharmacological DHEA administration seems to be suitable for patients with systemic lupus erythematosus and other related diseases."*

Adrenal-thyroid connection

Since I have just discussed cortisone and DHEA, which are both adrenal hormones, I thought it appropriate to examine the adrenal-thyroid connection because these two organs work together.

The thyroid is a butterfly-shaped gland situated at the base of the neck, just below the larynx, and is an endocrine gland, as it releases a hormone called thyroxine (T4) and small amounts of triiodothyronine (T3). T4 is an inactive pro-hormone. T3 is the active hormone. The inactive T4 is activated to T3 in the liver and in the peripheral tissues. The thyroid is regulated by thyroid-stimulating hormone (TSH) secreted by the pituitary gland. The pituitary is regulated by the part of the brain known as the hypothalamus. Thyroid hormone, specifically T3 completes the negative feedback loop as it has a negative effect on the release of TSH. The major function of thyroid hormone is to increase body metabolism.

When there is a low thyroid state, all organs, and tissues, including the adrenal glands are slowed down. Of course, the adrenal glands sensing this as a stressful situation try to keep up, but eventually the adrenal glands "fatigue." I use inverted commas because the adrenal gland does not "fatigue", although this is a commonly used term; it is the adrenal control mechanisms that become "fatigued."

With continued high stress and the constant release of cortisol, it is not that the adrenal "fatigues" or "tires out," rather a problem develops in the hypothalamus-pituitary-adrenal (HPA) axis. The HPA axis does not like the constant cortisol stimulation, so it *"switches off."*

Chronically elevated cortisol levels can cause damage, so the body tries to reduce the levels. The body tries to protect itself in several ways.

One way is by developing a cortisol receptor resistance.

Another way the body tries to protect itself from the high levels of cortisol is to increase the levels of cortisol binding globulin (CBG). This reduces the "free" cortisol by binding more (Chan, Carrell, Zhou, & Read, 2013; Mattos et al., 2013; Verhoog et al., 2014).

Another way to reduce the levels of cortisol is to convert the more active cortisol to the less active cortisone, by activation of *11 β-hydroxysteroid dehydrogenase type 2* (11β-HSD2).

Prigent, Maxime, and Annane (2003) showed that 11β-HSD2 can be upregulated by interleukins such as IL-2, IL-4 and IL-13. Maydych, Claus, Watzl, and Kleinsorge (2018) showed that interleukins are increased by stress and by inflammation.

In summary, most with "adrenal fatigue" do not necessarily have low cortisol levels. They may have low *"free"* cortisol levels but not necessarily low *"total"* cortisol levels.

Note that at least 80% of the cortisol is bound to corticosteroid binding globulin (CBG) and another 10% is bound to albumin. Only a small portion is unbound and therefore *"free,"* and only the *"free"* cortisol is biologically active. The low *"free"* cortisol produces the symptoms of low cortisol.

An "exhausted" adrenal gland does not produce less cortisol, but the regulatory mechanisms produce less *"free"* cortisol. There is also less DHEA, which can negatively influence the body.

Initially, when cortisol was measured using saliva, the low cortisol results gave the incorrect perception that the low cortisol measurement indicated the adrenal was not making the cortisol, that it was "fatigued." In reality, when saliva is used to measure cortisol, the result is that *"free"* cortisol is measured. There is a low *"free"* cortisol, not a low *"total"* cortisol.

Even if the thyroid is working normally, low *"free"* cortisol will eventually affect the whole thyroid system, not necessarily just at the hypothalamus and gland level, but also at the peripheral cellular level.

1) Stress with a consequent increase in endogenous cortisol secretion influences the hypothalamus, the thyroid gland itself and the body in general. There is a lowered TSH production, a blunted TSH response, a decline in T3 and an increased level of reverse T3 (rT3) (Rubello et al., 1992; Bános, Takó, Salamon, Györgyi, & Czikkely,1979).

2) When there is a high cortisol level, as in times of stress, T4 is more readily converted to rT3. Cortisol has a negative effect on the enzyme *5'deiodinase* (deiodinase type 2, DIO2) which converts T4 to T3: but has a positive action on another enzyme, *5 deiodinase* (deiodinase type 3, DIO3), which converts T4 to rT3. Reverse T3 (rT3) is a molecule structurally very similar to T3 but is inactive. Therefore, rT3 can act as a T3 blocker at the peripheral receptor sites or at least antagonise T3 (Okamoto & Leibfritz, 1997). Reverse T3 can inhibit T4 to T3 conversion (Chopra, 1977; Kelly, 2000).

215

To some extent this can be a protective mechanism. During times of stress, such as starvation, cold exposure, and so on, the body can protect itself by slowing down the metabolism to conserve energy (McCormack, Reed, Thomas, & Malik, 1996; Hackney, Feith, Pozos, & Seale, 1995).

3) T3 is needed at the mitochondrial level to produce cellular energy. However, both T3 and DHEA are needed at the mitochondrial level to work properly (Su & Lardy, 1991).

Therefore, if DHEA levels are low, which is common in "adrenal exhaustion," then the T3 will not work as well at the mitochondrial level.

As you can see, there is a close relationship between the thyroid gland and the adrenal glands. The function of one can significantly affect the other.

Stress was known in the past. Evolution developed a mechanism to deal with the short-term stress our ancestors had to deal with. This was the "fight or flight" response.

Chronic stress may have been an issue in the past, although it was not as prevalent, and not as widespread as it currently is. It has become a very big problem. Our physiology was not designed to deal with chronic stress, although our adrenal glands try hard to, and can manage to a certain degree. When the stress is prolonged, no organ can function indefinitely and "fatigue" sets in.

The changes in cortisol levels do not need to be huge. Even mild cortisol elevations within the normal physiological range seen during fasting, can suppress TSH.

"These results suggest that mild elevations in endogenous cortisol levels may mediate at least in part fasting-induced changes in TSH secretion and thyroid hormone levels. In addition, these data show that near-physiological doses of HC (hydrocortisone) and resulting changes in serum cortisol levels within the normal range can cause significant decreases in serum TSH levels" (Samuels & McDaniel, 1997).

Many people present with hypothyroid symptoms. They look clinically hypothyroid but have a normal TSH, as that is what most mainstream doctors check. They are not diagnosed with a thyroid problem but are fobbed off with a diagnosis such as "depression" and prescribed anti-depressants! See my previous book 'The Hypothyroid Syndrome' ISBN 978-0-6451053-3-9. The book can be ordered through any bookshop or online.

> If it looks like a duck, and walks like a duck, and quacks like a duck – it probably is a duck!

Those who present with hypothyroid symptoms may primarily have an adrenal issue and need adrenal treatment. Then, and only then, will their thyroid start to function normally. Another scenario is when a patient appears to be hypothyroid, but blood tests are mildly abnormal. The patient is commenced on thyroid replacement and becomes worse. It is important to look at the adrenal glands; they need to be treated primarily.

As stated earlier, modern medicine does not recognize "adrenal exhaustion" and, therefore, the treatment of this condition by conventional doctors is inadequate.

CONCLUSION

Hopefully by now you have a fuller understanding about hormones and how they affect human health. Also, by now you can see that hormones are very specific molecules, like a key that fits only a certain lock. You can also now see why the use of similar synthetics can cause so many health problems. The body was designed for the use of the exact hormone molecule, not something similar.

It is all too obvious why drug companies make similar molecule hormones; it is to circumvent the law about patenting natural molecules. Making profits by exploiting their product is another reason.

When drug companies or their paid agents say that the natural hormone is unsafe, consider it a warning and a nudge to do your own research. They have something to lose if their product is rejected: their business and their profits.

If you want better health, and you need to use a

hormone, then do not use synthetic similar analogues. Use the natural hormone.

The other half of this book is dedicated to a more clinical approach to the use of hormones. Hormonal issues are not necessarily only dealt with by simply replacing hormones. There are reasons why hormone balance goes awry. When the underlying issues are dealt with, and with proper nutrition and supplements, and even herbs, many issues will improve.

If hormones need to be supplemented, then only natural hormones and in physiological replacement doses should be used.

Part 2

INTRODUCTION

"Each progressive spirit is opposed by a thousand mediocre minds appointed to guard the past."

Maurice Maeterlinck (1863-1949)
Belgian playwright, poet, and essayist

"It takes 50 years to get a wrong idea out of medicine, and 100 years a right one into medicine."

John Hughlings Jackson (1835-1911)
British neurologist

Part 2 will focus mainly on the clinical aspects and treatment of hormone problems. I do not intend to focus only on bio-identical hormone replacement but will consider other aspects of hormone balance as well.

There is more to hormone balance than replacing hormones, even bioidentical. To simply replace what is considered to be missing makes the hormonal issue solely a deficiency disease and in some respects, this is not that much different from the mainstream view, which

223

is *"if there is a deficiency, then just replace what is missing."* Unquestionably, using bio-identical hormones (B-HRT) as replacement hormones is that much safer.

What the mainstream does not appreciate is that replacing hormones is not always the answer. The first half of the book gave the impression that hormone replacement is the only option: well, it isn't. We can do much more, but it does rely on the person to take some responsibility and make some life-style changes. The patient should be part of the solution and not part of the problem!

We must realise that as a person ages, hormone levels decline; this is part of the ageing programme. A healthy ageing person has fewer issues than does an unhealthy ageing person. We must focus on health, not just replace hormones.

Another perspective that is interesting to consider is whether we can keep a person young by continually replacing hormones?

Hormones seem to equal youth, after all, the young have higher levels and the old have lower levels. Therefore, it is not an unreasonable premise that keeping hormones at the "youthful level" keeps people young.

This is the thinking behind the advocates of the "anti-ageing" movement. They are not necessarily wrong; however, this method is not for everybody.

Some accept that "graceful ageing" is part of the great plan.

Others do not accept this and try to stay young for longer. We cannot live forever, and while hormone replacement is not exactly the "fountain of youth" in that it may not necessarily produce a *longer* life, it certainly can produce a better *quality* of life.

Simply replacing hormones may not always be the answer. We need to look at reasons why there are hormone imbalances in the first place.

One reason already alluded to is ageing itself. Organ function declines with age: an ageing brain will not release as many stimulating factors. An ageing gonad will not be able to manufacture the same amounts of hormone as a younger person's gonads. Certainly, from a sex hormone perspective, once the body has finished with the reproductive phase of life, there is no need for hormones to remain high, like in the younger age group. Simply replacing low hormones is not always good medicine.

We must treat the person as an individual who presents with symptoms. Not everyone with low hormones has a problem!

To some extent, *"If it ain't broke, don't fix it."*

As we age, a low level of hormones is the norm. We should not replace hormones just because they are low. We replace hormones because of symptoms.

However, before replacing hormones, we can give advice on healthy living, healthy eating and a healthy lifestyle, which can have an overall benefit.

On the other hand, at times, there may be no other way. The only way to treat some, is to supplement hormones.

> Everyone needs to be assessed individually. Not everyone with low hormones has a problem.

From a clinical point of view, we aim to treat the whole person. This includes their symptoms, and especially how they feel. It is important to look at the physical aspects, but the emotional, psychological, and even the spiritual aspects are equally important.

At one end of the spectrum, no hormones, supplements, herbs, or nutrition will alleviate a poor libido in a woman with a bad marriage. She would need counselling, psychological help - or a divorce lawyer!

Conversely, at the other extreme of the spectrum, a well, healthy, happy, confident woman, with no complaints, who is emotionally stable, and who has a great relationship but has low hormones, does not need to have her hormones treated.

There are many scenarios in-between!

There are three major philosophies for treating hormone issues.

First, there is the "anti-ageing" philosophy. This is where many hormones are supplemented to get the levels up to a "youthful" level. This is not necessarily because there are health issues, but because the levels are low. There may be an element of prevention, but the main idea is to keep hormone levels "youthful" so that there will be a better quality of life.

Second, at the other extreme, is the philosophy of not using any hormones at all but to look at the whole person and use exercise, diet, nutrients, lifestyle, and herbs to keep the person fit, well, and healthy. Hormones are not used in this case, not even the bio-identical ones.

There is a third philosophy. This is generally somewhere in between. Of course, diet, nutrition and lifestyle are used, but bio-identical hormones are used, judiciously. We must acknowledge that some people do need replacement hormones to function normally. Each person should be treated as an individual and tailor the treatment to their specific needs.

This is what I would advocate.

One group of people that would definitely need hormone replacement are those that have had surgical removal of gonads, either oophorectomy (removal of ovaries) in the woman or, in the man, orchidectomy (removal of testes).

We also must consider the philosophies of the person concerned. We could encourage them to change their diet and lifestyle, but some may not want to do this, they may just want a quick fix. Some may have already tried the diet, lifestyle, herbs, etc., which may not have worked to their satisfaction.

This may not be ideal, but it works, is safe, and the customer is satisfied! Then we have those with quite severe problems, where hormones may need to be used, even if only temporarily.

Then we have those who know what they want. They will seek a doctor who will satisfy their needs. I firmly believe that patients gravitate to the doctor who will treat them the way they would like to be treated. In today's world, people are more educated and more able to access information than ever before in the history of mankind. These well-informed men and women know what they want.

The patient chooses the doctor.

So, which is the correct method?

Perhaps they are all correct.

Let me put it another way: a person who wants the anti-ageing philosophy of treatment will gravitate to a doctor who practices that type of medicine.

People are attracted to a doctor based on their philosophy and how they want to be treated.

The patient chooses the doctor.

It is helpful to look at hormones and hormone balance from a diet and nutritional point of view. Eating the right diet can improve hormone balance. Nutrients also help, as do herbs and other natural products. One product does not fit all.

A body functions optimally only when fed correctly. Unfortunately, in today's modern world, very few people eat well. Many people eat the things that are advertised on TV and realistically, most of this is just junk with very little food value. This is not good eating. This is not scientific nutrition.

This is marketing.

The only science is in the psychology of advertising products to sell, so that the manufacturers can make profits.

Also, it is important to note that even if we do eat our meats, vegetables and salads, the quality of these foods is not great. The meat comes from animals that may have been pumped full of hormones, chemicals, and antibiotics. The animals are fed things that these animals generally do not eat. Cows are grass eaters; chickens eat grass and grubs and bugs and worms that they find from scratching around. This begs the question, why are they fed on grains, corn, and pellets, which are made from grain? This will alter the omega-3/omega-6 ratio, so that eating meat and eggs from animals fed in this way increases the omega-6 in our diet. Eating these animal products will increase the intake of the hormones, chemicals, and antibiotic residues. The best, and recommended, option is to buy grass-fed, free range, and organic meats.

Plant produce lacks many nutrients because of poor soil quality; this is especially so in Australia. The mineral content of any plant produce is determined by the mineral content of the soil. Commercial foods may have been sprayed with various chemicals, insecticides, herbicides, and pesticides, which leave behind multiple chemical residues.

For commercial purposes, many fruits are picked while still green and allowed to ripen in a box on the back of a truck while being transported to the other side of the country. Can we consider the fruit and vegetable ripened this way, healthy or wholesome? What about those products that are exposed to various chemicals to "ripen" them artificially? Or those products that are kept for months in the cool room? Can we truly consider them healthy or wholesome?

No, I don't think so!

If possible, to avoid fruit and vegetables that have no nutritional value, we should buy free-range, organic, and, where it is feasible, have the home veggie patch.

The home veggie patch has many advantages.

- To tend to the garden, you are outside in the sun, which will enhance your vitamin D levels.
- Gardening is an excellent form of exercise.
- Getting your hands dirty can build up immunity, and having your hands in the soil can be a good form of "grounding" – touch mother earth and feel the benefits of the experience.
- Gardening can relieve stress.
- Your harvested veggies are fresh and organic.
- There is also some food security, and your grocery bill will be lower.

If you are making your home veggie patch, make sure your soil is in tiptop condition: use lots of organic material, manure, and trace minerals. Then, and only then, will you have optimal healthy veggies.

Locally grown, seasonal produce is the best. Farmer's markets are a great way to get fresh local vegetables! At least when buying from such markets, the quality and the nutritional value are that much better than in what is bought from supermarkets.

Dietary change is an integral part of balancing hormones, as the wrong diet can upset the finely tuned balance of hormones.

As well as dietary considerations, there are other options, including nutrient supplementation and herbs, that should be considered before using B-HRT.

In this section, I will look at various hormonal conditions, including perimenopause, menopause, andropause, and a host of other conditions that are hormonally based. I will also outline the role of both nutrition and herbs in hormone balance, before exploring B-HRT use from a practical point of view.

PLEASE NOTE: I will not promote any specific product.

I will refer to vitamins and minerals and herbs as generics.

If a specific product is mentioned (e.g. as included in a quote), this is not necessarily an endorsement.

PRE-MENSTRUAL TENSION, PERI-MENOPAUSE AND MENOPAUSE

This chapter will concentrate on female hormone issues.

Premenstrual tension (PMT), also called premenstrual syndrome (PMS) in the USA, is a condition that occurs, as the name suggests, premenstrually, anything from two weeks to a few days before the onset of the period. It is regarded as a hormonal imbalance. As a rule of thumb, any symptom that presents before a period, or is aggravated before a period, is related to a relative oestrogen excess/progesterone deficiency.

Menopause refers to the period in a woman's life that signifies the end of the reproductive phase. The body has decided that the reproductive phase is over, so hormone levels decline. There is a male equivalent of menopause, commonly called andropause, and I will discuss that in the next chapter.

Premenstrual tension (PMT), which is called premenstrual syndrome (PMS), especially in the USA, refers to a range of physical and emotional symptoms that some women get in the second half of their menstrual cycle before their period starts. Many women will have some symptoms: in some they may be mild, while in others they can be very severe, resulting in discomfort and be distressing for a week or two every month. Symptoms start about four to fourteen days before a period and usually stop once bleeding begins. Symptoms can vary from woman to woman and may vary from one cycle to the next.

Perimenopause refers to the time from the onset of a change in menstrual cycle pattern or onset of menopausal symptoms, through to one year after the last menstrual period. The average duration is four to six years with onset in the fifth decade of life (40s).

Menopause refers to the final menstrual period and is said to have occurred when there have been no menstrual periods for one year. The average age of menopause in Australian women is 51 years (range 45-55 years).

Post-Menopause starts one year after the last menstrual period.

There is, in fact, a fairly fuzzy line between perimenopause, menopause, and post-menopause. For practical purposes, it is not always helpful to try to separate them. The line is artificial, and it is the person who should be treated, not the condition. The final period can only be known retrospectively!

The person should be treated and not the condition.

For treatment purposes, we should rely on the symptoms that each individual woman experiences. Treatment should be individualised, although there are many common patterns.

Symptoms of menopause

Symptoms are multiple and varied and can range from nil to extreme. One website lists 34 symptoms of menopause. Some may relate to female anatomy or function, some related to more emotional issues, but others are more general.

1) Hot flushes
2) Night sweats

3) Irregular periods

4) Mood changes

5) Breast soreness

6) Decreased libido

7) Vaginal dryness

8) Headaches

9) Recurring UTIs

10) Burning mouth

11) Changes in taste

12) Fatigue

13) Acne

14) Other digestive changes

15) Joint pain

16) Muscle tension and aches

17) Electric shock sensations

18) Itchiness

19) Sleep disturbance

20) Difficulty concentrating

21) Memory lapses

22) Thinning hair

23) Brittle nails

24) Weight gain

25) Stress incontinence

26) Dizzy spells

27) Allergies

28) Osteoporosis

29) Irregular heartbeat

30) Tinnitus

31) Irritability

32) Depression

33) Anxiety

34) Panic disorder

(https://www.medicalnewstoday.com › articles › what-are-the-34-symptoms-of-menopause)

One interesting symptom not mentioned in the above list is *formication* – no, not a typo! Formication from the Latin *formica* - ant. The sensation of ants crawling on the skin.

PMT symptoms

PMT is a condition, as the name implies, which occurs premenstrually, anything from two weeks to a few days before the onset of menses. The condition can range from mild and annoying to extremely severe.

There is a severe form of PMT, which may affect women at nearly all stages of life. The condition can be debilitating and is probably caused by extreme hormonal imbalances as well as other associated issues.

This condition should not be trivialised. It is a very serious issue; any woman with this extreme form of PMT is ready to kill. She needs as much help as we can administer.

Symptoms include:

- Moodiness, ranging from mild annoyance to uncontrollable rage, anger and aggression, which can be extreme.
- Heavy painful periods.
- Tiredness.
- Headaches and/or migraines.
- Breast swelling, lumpiness, soreness, nipple tenderness.
- Gut problems, bloating pain, constipation, or diarrhoea.
- Insomnia.
- Poor concentration.

Her husband/partner and all her colleagues, both male and female, stay well out of her way for certain days of the month. Even the dog knows when to steer clear! As mentioned above, this is a very serious condition and needs to be treated urgently. Not only is this severe form of PMT not conducive to a good relationship, but it also interferes with work and could even lead to criminal actions.

Premenstrual dysphoric disorder (PMDD)

I will mention this condition because some readers may have heard about it. This seems to be largely an American problem, which never caught on in Australia. Perhaps it is because of the difference in advertising laws.

What does a medical condition have to do with advertising laws?

Read on and find out.

Premenstrual dysphoric disorder (PMDD) is perhaps a bit of a ploy.

PMDD is defined as *"a health problem that is similar to premenstrual syndrome (PMS) but is more serious. PMDD causes severe irritability, depression, or anxiety in the week or two before your period starts. Symptoms usually go away two to three days after your period starts."*

241

(https://psychcentral.com/disorders/all-about-premenstrual-dysphoric-disorder)

Others have described it as being a "severe form of PMT."

(https://www.hopkinsmedicine.org/health/conditions-and-diseases/premenstrual-dysphoric-disorder-pmdd)

PMDD was "invented" and is not that much different from normal PMT, other than, in severity, only. In the USA, the Food and Drug Administration (FDA) has accepted PMDD as a separate condition, yet it does not seem to exist anywhere else in the world.

PMDD was advertised by the pharmaceutical companies as a distinct condition and then their drugs were heavily promoted as treatment. Some countries, such as USA and New Zealand can advertise medications directly to the public.

Advertisements appeared, such as *"Do you suffer from mood swings, irritability, insomnia, poor libido, etc, etc? Then you may have Premenstrual Dysphoric Disorder. Talk to your GP."* Of course, during this advertisement, the name of a drug is heavily promoted. So, what do women do? They go to their doctor and demand to be put on those drugs because they have this disease that was advertised on the TV. The GP also watches these same ads on TV and is "educated" to give the promoted drug. This is, of course, what the drug companies want. Make up a disease, or at least promote a set of symptoms, which may or may not be a disease, it could be just a part of life, then promote a drug and make $qillions in sales.

Other countries, including Australia, only allow companies to sponsor "disease awareness" campaigns.

The implication is that PMDD was invented for the purpose of medicalizing a condition, then promoting a drug to treat it. Whether it exists as a separate condition is debatable (Moynihan & Cassels, 2005; Fitzpatrick, 2005).

Many women suffer from PMT, however, there is a percentage of women who have an extreme form of this condition, which has been called PMDD. Medical conditions present as a spectrum from mild to severe. Could it be that PMDD is just a severe form of PMT?

Does it deserve a name of its own?

Just to clarify, I am only discussing this condition from a semantic point of view. Women with these severe symptoms need all the help they can get. They need all the treatment they can get, no matter what you call it.

I have really gone off the track!

Back to women's hormone issues.

Whether it is PMT, perimenopause or menopause, there are many symptoms and women suffering from the various symptoms, need help.

Often, these conditions are related to a "hormone imbalance." There can never be an imbalance if we consider only one hormone. There must be at least two.

Mainstream medicine seems to concentrate only on one, oestrogen. How can there be an imbalance of just one hormone? Excess or deficiency - yes - but not an imbalance.

Many of these hormonal disorders are not caused by an oestrogen deficiency but by an oestrogen-progesterone imbalance. We should primarily look at a progesterone deficiency.

We shouldn't look at absolute levels, but at a ratio. Mainstream medicine seems to focus mainly on oestrogen and only gives progestogens to prevent uterine cancer.

From personal clinical experience, oestrogen deficiency is not the most common problem, progesterone deficiency seems to be more common.

While the levels of oestrogen do decline, progesterone levels decline even more, almost to zero.

However, we need to be aware that there are many other oestrogens in our environment. We live in a sea of oestrogens, foreign compounds that have oestrogenic activity, which are commonly referred to as xenoestrogens. They may not necessarily have a steroidal structure like oestrogen, but they have oestrogenic activity, e.g. DES.

Xenoestrogens in our environment are largely derived from petrochemicals. They may be released as emissions, as in vehicle exhausts or factory emissions, or they may be in the products we use as insecticides, herbicides, plastics, dyes, drugs and cosmetics.

In this present time in history, petrochemicals are the basis of most manufacturing and therefore, are the cause of most of the pollution. Unfortunately, these products and their associated pollutants have xenoestrogenic properties, both oestrogenic and anti-oestrogenic effects. They are often called "gender-benders" because of the havoc they can play on our finely tuned hormonal system.

When blood oestrogen levels are measured, we can only measure the natural endogenous oestrogen in that person. In fact, if we measure oestrogen in the blood, we can only detect what is floating in the blood, as most of the hormone is intracellular, it cannot be determined by blood tests. This will be discussed later. We can only speculate on the level of exogenous oestrogens present. Despite not being able to be measured easily, they have an impact.

The total body exposure to oestrogens is the sum total of the external xenoestrogens plus the endogenously produced oestrogens. The blood tests may show low oestrogen, but there may be an overall oestrogen excess.

For this reason, a large majority of women are oestrogen dominant. They have too much oestrogen in relation to progesterone and so are (relatively) progesterone deficient.

Hormone testing

Testing of hormones can be useful before commencing treatment. The mainstream relies on blood hormone measurements, whereas integrative and alternative doctors often use salivary hormone testing.

How useful are these measurements?

What are the pros and cons?

Salivary versus serum?

This is usually a controversial issue.

Let's start with some basics.

Steroid hormones are derived from cholesterol, they are lipophilic, that is, basically fats. How can you expect to measure a fatty substance in the watery part of the blood?

Water and oil do not mix.

One assumption is that the hormones we measure in the serum represent the hormones in the whole blood. Can this measurement be accurate if approximately half of whole blood is serum, and the rest comprises blood cells? This assumes that the blood cells play no role in hormone transport.

This is not so.

Approximately 80% of progesterone is carried by the red blood cells (RBC) (Koefoed & Brahm, 1994), and so these cells play an important role in hormone transport.

This is one reason there is a discrepancy between the serum progesterone and the salivary progesterone: eighty percent is removed when the blood is spun down to separate the serum from the blood cells.

Topical progesterone can increase tissue levels of progesterone without necessarily increasing serum levels.

Not only do RBC carry progesterone, but they can carry other steroids as well.

Another assumption is that the amount of hormone measured in the serum reflects the actual level of active hormone in the tissues.

However, this assumption is not correct.

Why saliva?

Saliva forms in the salivary glands by electrolytes being actively pumped in. Water follows by osmosis. Blood components, including IgA, IgG, and *"free"* hormones (that is hormones not bound to the binding proteins) diffuse freely into the saliva.

Therefore, the level of hormones in the saliva is a measure of the *"free"*, unbound hormone that is found intracellularly. This is important because the actions of hormones are intracellular. The steroid hormone receptors are intracellular. It is important to know how much hormone is in the cells, not necessarily what is floating in the blood. This is like examining the content of a truck on a highway and determining the level of stores in the warehouse and/or the factory.

One paradox is that when topical hormones are used, the salivary level is very much higher than the serum level. This paradox perturbs mainstream practitioners, and they dismiss the whole notion of salivary testing. They believe their blood testing is the gold standard that all things should be measured against.

Could it be that the serum levels are the problem?

Chang, Lee, Linares-Cruz, Fournier, and de Ligniéres (1995) looked at oestrogen and progesterone cream rubbed into breast skin in women prior to benign breast lump surgery. They showed an increase in breast tissue hormone levels without a concomitant serum level increase.

Many mainstream doctors do not believe in topical progesterone because it does not increase serum levels. This is largely due to errors in the mainstream measurement methods. They are examining the wrong part of the blood.

The advantages of salivary hormone testing are that it is:

1) Easier,
2) Less traumatic,

3) Can be done at home,
4) The specimen is stable and allows for convenient shipment,
5) Serum levels can fluctuate more widely than salivary samples,
6) Multiple samples can be easily taken.

The disadvantages of salivary testing are:

1) It is technically more difficult because of the very small amount needed to be measured,
2) Salivary hormone testing is carried out by only a few specialised laboratories, so accreditation is required, and standards must be maintained,
3) Food and drinks such as coffee can interfere with results,
4) Contamination can occur, especially if a troche* is used, or even from a person's hand after applying B-HRT cream.
5) Cost: serum blood tests are covered by Medicare, but salivary hormones are not.

* Troche: a means of giving hormones. A troche is like a lozenge and is slowly dissolved under the tongue or between the gum and cheeks, allowing for absorption through the oral mucosa.

Here I diverge with an interesting anecdote. I measured salivary hormones in a gentleman whose results were very unusual. He had an extremely high progesterone level. I was wracking my brain trying to work out why. Then I realised. His wife was using progesterone troches, and there was the possibility that there must have been some saliva exchange at some point!

Gröschl (2008) was very positive about salivary hormone testing. *"Although saliva has not yet become a mainstream sample source for hormone analysis, it has proven to be reliable and, in some cases, even superior to other body fluids. Nevertheless, much effort will be required for this approach to receive acceptance over the long term, especially by clinicians. Such effort includes the development of specific and standardized analytical tools, the establishment of defined reference intervals, and implementation of round-robin trials. One major problem, the lack of compliance sometimes seen in outpatient saliva donors, requires strict standardization of both collection and analysis methods to achieve better comparability and assessment of published salivary hormone data."*

So, what do I do? Lately, I mostly do serum hormone levels because of the current economic climate. Many can barely afford to see the doctor, let alone pay extra for salivary hormone testing.

With hormone blood tests, I do take the above factors into consideration.

Do we have to test hormones? Initially, it may be a good idea, just to get a full picture. Some have asked: "How can you treat what you cannot measure?" "Can you treat hypertension without measuring blood pressure?" "Can you treat diabetes without measuring BSL?"

There is the argument that we can use our clinical judgement. Certainly, once treatment has started, we can monitor the patient just by asking, *"How do you feel?"*

If the person says that they are feeling terrific, then we know to a great degree of certainty, that their hormone balance must be good.

Hormone levels may still be worth measuring intermittently.

Why, if the person is feeling well?

Possibly for medico-legal reasons. If you are supplementing a hormone, I believe it is good practice to monitor it.

However, before we even consider supplementing hormones, we should take a good history and assess each person individually. We should look at things like diet, nutrition, health, fitness, associated illnesses, as these can all have an impact.

The hot flush

Note to any American readers: a hot flush is the same as a hot flash!

The hot flush is possibly the most exasperating symptom of menopause; in fact, it is the symptom most associated with the menopause. The hot flush, as the name implies, is a sudden onset of heat, usually in the upper part of the body, and can range from a mild sensation of heat to a raging inferno associated with saturating sweats. When they occur at night, they are obviously called "night sweats" and again can range from mild clamminess to severe drenching, to the extent that nighties and bed sheets need to be changed.

The question often asked is: "What causes these hot flushes?"

The answer is: "Nobody knows for sure."

Much is known about the hot flush. While there are many ideas, the definitive cause is not known for sure, although possibly it is multi-factorial.

It has something to do with hormone imbalance and something to do with the hypothalamus. We know that the hormone monitoring part of the hypothalamus is next door to the vaso-motor centre (the part of the brain that controls arterial and venous dilatation). Therefore, we can speculate that if the hormone monitoring centre is over-active, some action will diffuse to the nearby vaso-motor centre, making the body's thermostat more sensitive, more unstable, to changes in body temperature.

The research is contradictory!

Freedman, Norton, Woodward, and Cornélissen (1995) studied core temperatures of symptomatic and asymptomatic women. The researchers found the core body temperature to be lower in symptomatic women than asymptomatic women, but there is a rise in core temperature preceding a flush.

However, in a newer study, Freedman (2002) measured core temperature with an ingested radiotelemetry pill in three groups of women,

1) symptomatic postmenopausal women who had a hot flush in the laboratory,

2) symptomatic postmenopausal women who did not have a flush in the laboratory, and

3) asymptomatic postmenopausal women.

No significant differences were found among the three groups.

Most of the heat seems to come from peripheral vasodilation, that is, the veins in the skin dilate to give off the heat. There is some evidence that there is a minor elevation of core temperature that triggers the hot flush (Freedman, 2014).

Despite these measurements and a lot of research, the actual cause is still not known.

We know that as the woman ages, the oestrogen level declines, and many have considered this to be the definite cause. After all, supplementing oestrogen relieves the flushes. Yet, this is not the full story because supplementing progesterone alone can also relieve the flushes.

Conversely, some women with low hormones do not have flushes, so the oestrogen relationship is not that clear.

An interesting fact is that in some cases, hot flushes can occur with high oestrogen levels (oestrogen dominance). Progesterone can relieve hot flushes by balancing the oestrogen dominance. Di indolyl methane (DIM) or indole 3 carbinol (I3C), which are broccoli extracts, can reduce hot flushes in this situation by lowering oestrogen levels. This reduction of oestrogen levels improves the oestrogen/progesterone balance.

Men can also suffer from hot flushes, especially if being treated with anti-androgen therapy, or if they have had an orchidectomy (removal of testes).

Hot Flushes are worse in more obese women (Koo, Ahn, Lim, Cho, & Park, 2017), smokers (Cochran, Gallicchio, Miller, Zacur, & Flaws, 2008) and women who exercise more, have fewer flushes (Bailey et al., 2016).

There is more to hot flushes than sex hormones.

Other hormones have also been implicated.

"Serum leptin levels are associated with the occurrence and duration of hot flashes in midlife women; however, no correlation was found between leptin and serum estradiol" (Alexander et al., 2010).

So here we can see that it is not strictly sex hormone levels that are important; other hormones are implicated. Leptin is a hormone closely related to obesity and to lifestyle. Insulin has also been implicated.

Some non-hormonal factors have also been associated with hot flushes.

Martin, Block, Sanchez, Arnaud, and Beyene (1993) researched the Mayan women of Yucatan, Mexico. They showed a similar oestrogen decline as seen in western women, but without the symptoms. The researchers were forced to admit that menopausal symptoms are not necessarily related to oestrogen decrease only. The researchers could not elicit any history of hot flushes and despite living to an age 30 years past menopause, no increase in osteoporosis was found. These women, had more babies, hardly ever used contraception and their emotional state was much different. Age is respected and as these women get older, they are elevated into a higher status amongst her people. They also live in a cleaner, non-polluted environment.

A similar view can be concluded from the studies of Professor Margaret Lock, a medical anthropologist from McGill University. She conducted a study on Japanese menopausal women and found that the Japanese lifestyle, as well as their attitude to menopause, plays a very important protective role (Lock, 1998).

Japanese women have the world's highest life expectancy, and a much lower rate of breast cancer, heart disease and osteoporosis than western women. They also have very few menopausal symptoms as compared to western women. Only about 20% of women complain about hot flushes, compare this to approximately 60% of western women. The traditional Japanese diet, which is high in fish, vegetables and soy, is probably a contributing factor.

The Mayan and Japanese women view menopause differently from western women. These women have a positive attitude to age, as age is respected in their cultures. In the west, there is an anti-ageing attitude. Youth is 'in' and age is 'out'. This gives a very negative attitude to menopause. As you can see, there is a large sociological aspect to menopause.

A study called the Women's Midlife Health Project examined these same factors. They found that "negative attitudes to ageing or menopause were consistently associated with more symptoms."

"Analysis of variance of factor scores found fewer symptoms with increasing years of education, better self-rated health, the use of fewer non-prescription medications, the absence of chronic health conditions, a low level of interpersonal stress, the absence of premenstrual complaints, not currently smoking, exercise at least once a week, and positive attitudes to ageing and menopause" (Dennerstein et al. 1993).

So, it's not just hormones, diet, and lifestyle. Culture, attitude and expectations also play a role in this multi-factorial phenomenon.

Let's have a look at some of these lifestyle and diet factors.

Obese women have more hot flushes (Koo, Ahn, Lim, Cho, & Park, 2017). Losing weight has been shown to reduce the incidence and intensity of hot flushes (Huang et al., 2010).

In a study by Yokota, Makita, Hirasawa, Iwata, and Aoki (2016), 1,969 Japanese women aged 40 to 60 years were classified into three groups,

1) low BMI (under-weight),

2) normal BMI (normal weight), and

3) high BMI (over-weight).

Researchers found that the most common symptom was general fatigue. The researchers also found that the incidence of hot flushes, sweats, joint pain, numbness, and incontinence was higher in the over-weight group. The underweight group had significantly more severity of cold constitution, nervousness, and wrinkled skin. They also showed that an increase in body weight increased the incidence of vasomotor symptoms.

Why would this be a cause?

Obesity is related to high insulin levels. There is a connection between high insulin and sex hormone binding globulin (SHBG). The higher the insulin, the lower the SHBG. Dietary sugar itself can reduce the liver's ability to make SHBG (Selva, Hogeveen, Innis, & Hammond, 2007).

We also know that if the SHBG is low, there is a much higher level of "free" testosterone.

So what?

At least one study has shown that hot flushes are related to elevated testosterone levels. *"Women with hot flushes had higher testosterone and FTI (Free Testosterone Index) and women reporting coldness had lower concentrations"* (Gotmar et al., 2008).

Then there is the increased level of *aromatase* in the obese. *Aromatase* is largely in the fat cells, therefore, if there are more fat cells, then there is more *aromatase*. *Aromatase* is an enzyme that converts testosterone to oestrogen. High levels of *aromatase* in obese men convert testosterone to oestrogen, which is not a good thing for men. This is a cause for the "man boobs" / "moobs" that we can see on many men. Zinc is a good *aromatase* inhibitor, another good reason for men to take extra zinc. Dose of zinc: 15-30 mgs, zinc daily.

Supplement zinc in males.

Insulin inhibits *aromatase*. Lower levels seem to stimulate *aromatase* action, while higher insulin levels inhibit it (Bhatia & Price, 2001).

In women with high insulin levels, testosterone is not converted to oestrogen, which leads to a higher testosterone level, which is not a good thing for women.

So, the high sugar and carbohydrate diet is related to higher insulin levels and obesity, and this can increase levels of testosterone, which has a relationship to hot flushes.

Other hot flush triggers

There are other triggers that can cause hot flushes.

One of the most common is stress.

Stress and hot flushes are related. Women who are more stressed have more hot flushes. But then, more hot flushes can cause more stress.

Is this a psychological issue or a physiological issue? We do know that stress causes the release of adrenaline, noradrenaline and cortisol, which can cause palpitations and hot flushes.

Have you ever had a near-miss car accident or some other similar scary event? Did you get a hot flush? Does this release of stress hormones cause the flush? Again, the answer is not so simple.

Tulandi, Murphy, and Lal (1985) did *not* show any increase in cortisol secretion in women with frequent hot flushes.

However, Woods, Carr, Tao, Taylor, and Mitchell (2006) did show a relationship. *"Increased cortisol levels during the late MT (Menopausal Transition) stage, when menstrual irregularities are greatest, suggests increases in adrenal androgens and intraabdominal fat with menopause, and may influence risk of cardiovascular disease, vasomotor symptoms, mood, cognition, and bone loss."*

This has been confirmed by a more recent study (Woods, Mitchell, & Smith-Dijulio, 2009).

Stress must have a role in the causation of the hot flush because psychological methods to reduce stress can treat hot flushes (Kagan & Dusek, 2006). Yoga has also been shown to reduce menopausal symptoms

(Chattha, Raghuram, Venkatram, & Hongasandra, 2008). Acupuncture and applied relaxation also show benefit (Zaborowska et al., 2007).

In one study, exercise was observed to cause hot flushes. This study looked at "highly active women" compared to "minimally active women" (Whitcomb, Whiteman, Langenberg, Flaws, & Romani, 2007).

In another study (Nelson et al., 2008) showed exercise to have multiple beneficial effects in the improvement of anxiety, stress, and depression, but there was no association between levels of physical activity and hot flushes.

So, which is it? Is exercise good or bad for hot flushes? A third study (Romani, Gallicchio, & Flaws, 2009) concluded that higher levels of physical activity were associated with *"increasing odds of moderate or severe hot flashes".*

However, Bailey et al. (2016) wrote, *"Exercise training that improves cardiorespiratory fitness reduces self-reported hot flushes."*

Exercise, then, is important for health, but it should be moderate exercise … not too much … not too little; the "Goldilocks' zone".

McCallum and Reading (1989) showed that being

too hot, eating hot foods, spicy foods, drinking hot drinks, being in a hot environment, over-heating the house, being too warm under the doona, even over-dressing can all be a cause of a hot flush; any thermogenic stimulus can induce a hot flush. The vasomotor centre appears to become more unstable, more "irritable", so that even a minor increase in temperature can trigger a flush.

Sievert et al. (2002) suggest a few things that can be related to hot flushes. While drinking coffee, and variables such as room temperature are possibly well-known potential triggers of a hot flush, others such as months spent breast feeding the last child, and the weight you were at age 18, are not so well known.

Another cause is drugs.

There are many drugs used by women, which have side effects of hot flushes, increased sweating, and vasodilatation.

These include anti-hypertensive drugs (e.g. verapamil, nifedipine, amlodipine), anti-depressant drugs (selective serotonin reuptake inhibitors (SSRIs) e.g. sertraline, fluoxetine, paroxetine), various hormone-mimic drugs (e.g. tamoxifen, raloxifene), steroids, opiates, tricyclic antidepressants, clomiphene, and MAO inhibitors. Consider how many menopausal women could be on some of these drugs.

This highlights an interesting point; how ironic it is that some advocate the use of anti-depressants to treat hot flushes when one of the side effects *is* hot flushes!

When did this trend of using antidepressants for hot flushes start? Why would the use of an antidepressant drug even be considered to treat hot flushes?

This trend started soon after the release of the Women's Health Initiative (WHI) study, the time when hundreds of thousands of women all over the world threw their HRT into the bin. SSRIs were considered because various studies showed that some women on these drugs seemed to have fewer hot flushes, or at least complained less. Could it be that the women on anti-depressants just "didn't care" about the hot flushes and did not complain? Anti-depressants cause emotional blunting; therefore, user's emotions are dulled, and they no longer feel strong emotions. *"I have a hot flush ... but who cares?"*

Some studies were positive.

"Sertraline to treat hot flashes: a randomised, double-blind, crossover trial in a general population" (Gordon, Kerwin, Boesen, & Senf, 2006).

"Paroxetine controlled release in the treatment of menopausal hot flashes: a randomised controlled trial" (Stearns, Beebe, Iyengar, & Dube, 2003).

Other studies show **no** benefit.

"Ineffectiveness of sertraline for treatment of menopausal hot flushes: a randomised controlled trial" (Grady et al., 2007).

"Citalopram and fluoxetine in the study of postmenopausal symptoms: a prospective randomised, 9-month, placebo-controlled, double-blind study" (Suvanto-Luukkonen et al., 2005).

Also, in a study where the antidepressant fluoxetine was compared with the herb black cohosh (*Actaea racemosa*, also called *Cimicifuga racemosa*) the researchers found that black cohosh was *more* effective in treating hot flushes and night sweats. Fluoxetine was more effective in treating depression (Oktem et al., 2007).

Breast problems

Most breast disorders, including cancer, are caused by, or closely related to. hormone imbalances, which may either be a relative or an absolute excess of oestrogen in relation to progesterone. Oestrogen can be considered the accelerator, while progesterone can be considered the brake. Therefore, to treat these conditions, we have to balance the hormones, either by reducing the oestrogen, or by increasing the progesterone, or perhaps both.

Breast symptoms are a very common complaint in women, especially during times of hormonal fluctuation, such as pregnancy, PMT and menopause. These symptoms are also seen in women who are on oestrogen only HRT and many do complain bitterly about their sore swollen breasts.

Symptoms include breast swelling, soreness, lumpiness, sensitive nipples, sensitivity to touch and/or a dull heavy sensation.

Since the breast symptoms are caused by hormonal fluctuations, many of the herbs and nutrients that are discussed in this book that alter oestrogen metabolism can be also treat breast problems.

Some women develop lumps, and these always, not unreasonably, cause fear, because of the concern about breast cancer.

A painful lump is less likely to be cancerous; it is more likely to be a hormone imbalance produced lump. Such lumps wax and wane, being especially more prominent before a period. Any lump that is fixed, hard, and non-tender *needs* to be investigated to the full extent with ultrasound, a mammogram, and biopsy.

MRI is now being advocated instead of a mammogram because no radiation is involved. There is a possible link between radiation and cancer.

One should not rely on the fact that a lump is or is not tender/painful. *Any* lump needs to be taken seriously and investigated fully until proven to be cancerous or non-cancerous.

A lump proven not to be cancerous can be treated with the herbs and nutrients mentioned in this book. There are some specific nutrients that are beneficial for the breast.

A sore lumpy breast diagnosed as fibrocystic breast disease (FBD) responds well to iodine supplementation (Ghent, Eskin, Low, & Hill, 1993).

Vitamin A has been shown to have positive results in the treatment of benign breast disease (Band, Deschamps, Falardeau, Ladouceur, & Cote, 1984) and possibly breast cancer (Kim, Jang, & Lee, 2021).

Mirzaee, Fakari, Babakhanian, Roozbeh, and Ghazanfarpour (2022) stated that pharmaceuticals such as danazol and bromocriptine are used to treat the monthly breast symptoms that many women have prior to their periods. These drugs do have side effects, so many would prefer herbal medicines. The researchers looked at various herbs and nutrients: Vitex agnus-castus, flaxseed, evening primrose oil, chamomile, isoflavone, cinnamon and Nigella sativa, and all were helpful in relieving mastalgia.

On the positive side, these nutrients can be used safely, especially when the orthodox treatment involves the use of drugs or surgery.

There is evidence that the removal of methyl-xanthenes, contained in coffee, tea, chocolate, and cola drinks, may be beneficial, especially with fibrocystic breast disease (La Vecchia et al., 1985; Minton, Abou-Issa, Reiches, & Roseman, 1981).

Again, there are conflicting results, but on the positive side, it is safe to eliminate these products from the diet and see if this works for you.

Many breast problems are related to oestrogen imbalances.

Liver support herbs, such as St Mary's thistle (*Silybum marianum*), can be useful, because of the liver's role in oestrogen metabolism. Bowel function needs to be improved as constipation has been shown to aggravate oestrogen dependant breast problems.

Herbs, such as Angelica sinensis (dong quai), and Vitex agnus-castus, can be helpful as they influence hormone metabolism. Indole 3 carbinol (I3C) and di indolyl methane (DIM) which are both broccoli extracts, can also be used.

A specific herb that is used traditionally for breast problems is Phytolacca (*Phytolacca dioica, Phytolacca americana and Phytolacca decandra*), either as a homeopathic remedy, a poultice or as a cream to be applied topically. The success is based mainly on traditional and/or anecdotal evidence.

Bailly (2021) showed that there are *"... various types of Phytolacca extracts, showing a range of pharmacological activities including antioxidant, anti-inflammatory, anti-parasitic, antifungal, anticancer, and insecticidal effects."*

Phytolacca as a cream or in a homeopathic form is certainly worth trying.

B-HRT can also treat breast conditions as this is a part of treating the whole woman. More often than not, women do *not* need extra oestrogen, they only need progesterone replacement.

Hormone balance and diet

Perhaps the best place to start is with the diet. Dietary change can help not only hormonal issues but many other chronic health problems as well. Primitive tribes living and eating in their natural environment do not have many of the hormonal and chronic health issues that we have in the west. They may have other significant health problems, but that is not the subject of this book.

Once "western civilization" arrives, and people start to eat and live like the "white man," disease soon follows.

So, the big question here is: *"What is the best diet for women (or men) with hormonal problems, or for any other health issue, for that matter?"*

We can look to the "low stress diet" (LSD). This diet, as the name implies, is "low stress," and minimises the burden placed on the body. The diet, or rather, an "eating pattern," is low in refined and processed foods, bread, pasta, cereals, sugar, dairy, coffee, chocolate, alcohol, or anything coming from a factory. This eating pattern would also avoid additives, colourings, flavourings, and preservatives.

This eating pattern is high in essential nutrients

and includes vegetables, legumes, meats, eggs, nuts, seeds, and fruits. Fresh and organic is, of course, the best. We can use the mnemonic SLOW (Seasonal Local Organic Whole). This eating pattern is approximating our ancestral diet - the "cave man diet" if you will. We should eat the diet we evolved with, the diet our physiology evolved with and adapted to, and not the diet of the civilized western society, which is a novel concept, and to which our physiology has not yet adapted. The LSD will provide many essential nutrients, as well as reducing the stress on the gut and the liver. This is important because these two systems are involved greatly in hormonal balance.

"It is widely accepted that diet and lifestyle play a large part in symptom relief and evidence is strengthening for the role of phytoestrogens in the relief of hot flushes" (Jefferson, 2005).

Nutrients

Hormones are made by a series of steps converting one molecule to another, in a regular order. These steps are controlled by various enzymes which need co-factors to work. In many cases, these co-factors are vitamins and/or minerals.

One of the basic principles of nutritional medicine is to supplement raw materials, co-factors, vitamins, and minerals to encourage these biochemical steps. If you know the biochemistry, then you know what vitamin or mineral to supplement to help the reaction along.

Nutritional Medicine is Applied Biochemistry.

Clearly, if there is a specific nutrient missing, then one or more of the biochemical steps are likely to be affected.

For example, the first step in the steroid pathway is the conversion of cholesterol to pregnenolone, which is achieved by a cytochrome P 450 enzyme (CPY 11A1) in the inner membrane of the adrenocortical mitochondria (Ohta et al., 1990). This reaction is dependent on an NADP/NADPH (nicotinamide adenine dinucleotide phosphate) reaction which requires magnesium. NADP is a derivative of vitamin B3 (niacin). This means that if there is a magnesium and vitamin B3 deficiency, the first step in hormone synthesis may be affected.

For the body to convert cholesterol to oestrogen,

273

progesterone, and DHEA, a full complement of vitamins and minerals is needed. An analogy would be trying to build a house. You may have the bricks, the cement, and the lime, but if the sand is missing, can you then build your house? No, of course not. If you made the attempt, quality would be poor, bits would be missing, and it would probably fall apart quickly.

It is the same with the body. If one nutrient, that is, one co-factor, is missing, some biochemical steps will be disrupted.

Why am I saying this? Mainly because the level of nutrition in many parts of the world is extremely poor. Third-world countries are malnourished by being under-fed because of a lack of any food.

"Civilized" western countries are over-fed yet are still malnourished. Most foods consumed by most people are highly refined and processed in factories; they therefore become nutrient deficient. Even if fresh foods are eaten, many nutrients are missing due to poor farming practices and poor soil quality. Many people living in western countries are nutrient deficient. The deficiency of just one nutrient could interfere with many pathways. A deficiency of several nutrients can cause an even greater amount of disruption.

Another scenario is where there may be toxic

heavy metals (HMs) such as lead, mercury, cadmium, aluminium, and so on present. Who, in this polluted western society, does not have HMs in their body? HMs act as "anti-nutrients" and can block the action of many nutrients with the result being a situation mimicking a nutritional deficiency.

The major nutrients needed are magnesium, zinc, iron, the B vitamins, and vitamin C.

Encouraging a diet high in these nutrients or supplementing them will encourage the biochemical reactions in all systems as well as the production of the sex hormones.

A good source of zinc is meat of any sort. Vegetarians tend to be zinc deficient. Magnesium comes from green leafy vegetables, but only when there is adequate magnesium in the soil. Vitamin C degrades very easily and, therefore, is only found in fresh (straight off the tree or from the garden) fruits and vegetables. B12 only comes from animal sources and therefore is deficient in vegetarians and vegans.

Many other nutrients are removed or destroyed during food processing.

When you know what most westerners eat, you should not be too surprised at the level of nutritional deficiency!

Phytoestrogens

Phytoestrogens are sometimes referred to as "dietary oestrogens", yet this term is, in fact, a misnomer. They should be called "phytosterols" because these molecules are not specifically oestrogenic. They can bind to all steroid receptors. So, from here on, I will refer to them as phytosterols.

Phytosterols are a diverse group of naturally occurring non-steroidal plant compounds (lignans, coumestans, isoflavones and resorcylic acid) which have some structural similarity to the steroidal hormones. They have the ability to cause hormonal and/or anti-hormone effects because they can interact with the steroid receptor. These compounds are specifically used because they are thought to interact with the oestrogen receptor.

Phytosterols can be found in virtually every food we eat, specifically fresh foods (note that refined foods have a lower content). A good daily intake can be beneficial.

Foods high in phytosterols include: soybeans, tofu, tempeh, soy beverages, linseed (flax), sesame seeds, wheat, berries, oats, barley, dried beans, lentils, yams, rice, alfalfa, mung beans, apples, carrots, garlic, squash, green beans, broccoli, cabbage, nuts, fruits, berries, pomegranates, wheat germ, rice-bran, ginseng, bourbon, beer, fennel and anise.

However, there are some people who may react adversely to some of the above foods. For example, some may react to the gluten in the grains.

Although vegans/vegetarians may be low in some minerals, especially zinc, Beezhold, Radnitz, McGrath, and Feldman (2018) showed that vegans reported fewer vasomotor and physical symptoms than omnivores. This is more than likely due to the increased intake of phytosterols in the diet.

Plants that are outstandingly high in phytosterols can be considered medicinal herbs. Some examples are black cohosh, chaste tree berry, dong quai, ginseng, liquorice, sage, fenugreek, saw palmetto and wild yam root. Many readers will recognize at least some of these herbs as they have been used in traditional herbal practice for a very long time.

For a while, the flavour of the month was soy. Soy was touted to reduce or eliminate many of the symptoms of hot flushes and other menopausal symptoms. We know that there are various phytosterols, such as *genistein* and *daidzein* in soy, and theoretically, they are the reason soy may help. However, the research shows conflicting evidence. Some studies gave negative results, while others showed positive outcomes (Imhof, Gocan, Imhof, & Schmidt, 2018; Faure, Chantre & Mares, 2002).

What about herbs?

I know herbs work because I have seen it so many times in my practice.

Kargozar, Azizi, and Salari (2017) studied various herbs and wrote that *"The results of the study showed that the medicinal plants, which include Sage herb (Salvia officinalis), Lemon balm (Melissa officinalis), Valerina officinalis, Black cohosh (Cimicifuga racemosa), Fenugreek (Trigonella foenum-graecum), Black cumin (Nigella sativa), Vitex (Vitex agnus-castus), Fennel (Foeniculum vulgare), Evening primrose (Oenothera biennis), Ginkgo biloba, Alfalfa (Medicago sativa), Hypericum perforatum, Panax ginseng, Pimpinella anisum, Licorice (Glycyrrhiza glabra), Passiflora incarnata, Red clover (Trifolium pratense), and Glycine soja were effective in the treatment of acute menopausal syndrome (which includes hot flushes) with different mechanisms."*

Many living in a western society have a poor diet that consists of mainly processed foods that contain very few phytosterols. Additionally, many have poor gut function and suffer from dysbiosis (excess of "bad" bacteria in the gut), which may interfere with the action of phytosterols (Leonard, Choi & Cross, 2022).

A healthy gut microbiome is necessary for proper utilisation of phytosterols. This is certainly one reason why soy, or some herbs, do not work for all.

Treatment for poor digestion and dysbiosis is by supplementing probiotics and other gut supporting measures.

Support the gut.

Sugar and refined carbohydrates

Some of the worst food offenders for producing poor health, obesity and other diseases of western civilization are sugars and other refined carbohydrates.

Studies have shown that hot flushes are related to blood sugar levels (BSL). Dormire and Reame (2003) infused subjects with either glucose or saline. The researchers found a significant reduction in hot flushes while the BSL was high than when the BSL was low.

In a later study, Dormire and Howharm (2007) agreed with their earlier research; hot flush frequency is suppressed after eating, while hot flushes are experienced when BSL falls.

I think we can extrapolate from these studies that a refined carbohydrate, high sugar intake (typical of western diets) can cause an unstable BSL and can trigger hot flushes.

Having a high carbohydrate, sugary snack before bedtime could lead to a hypoglycaemic attack in the middle of the night. One of the symptoms of hypoglycaemia is sweating, which can be interpreted as a hot flush.

A highly refined, sugary diet leads to hyperinsulinaemia and secondary insulin resistance; this sets the scene for reactive hypoglycaemic attacks. Low BSL trigger hot flushes.

We have mentioned before that obesity is related to hot flushes, and losing weight can reduce them. A higher protein, lower carbohydrate, sugar-free diet helps to reduce obesity.

A high sugar and refined carbohydrate diet (the typical western diet) elevates insulin levels. High insulin levels reduce the SHBG. SHBG is the protein that binds the sex hormones, therefore, when the hormone is bound, it is inactive.

Only the unbound, "free" hormone has biological activity. When there are low SHBG levels, there are fewer binding sites, therefore, "free" testosterone rises. As we have already seen, women with higher testosterone levels have more hot flushes.

If sugar and refined carbohydrates are reduced in the diet, insulin levels will drop, which will increase the SHBG, which binds more "free" testosterone, which will reduce the hot flushes.

Berrino et al. (2001) showed that a diet *"low in animal fat and refined carbohydrates and rich in low-glycemic-index foods, monounsaturated and n-3 polyunsaturated fatty acids, and phytoestrogens"* can reduce IR and increase SHBG and reduce testosterone in hyperandrogenic women.

Now you can see why women who are obese and who exercise less have more hot flushes.

Treatment of Menopausal Symptoms and Hot Flushes includes:

1) Reduce sugars and refined carbohydrates in the diet

2) Increase exercise, but not too much

3) Reduce alcohol intake

4) Reduce stress... learn to relax.

5) Stop smoking

6) Lose weight

7) Keep cool.

Liver support

Earlier on, I touched on the topic of liver function and its role in hormone metabolism. The ovaries (and adrenal glands) make the hormones, but it is the liver that metabolises and eliminates them. The liver cannot actually break down these hormones, but it can make them less active and more soluble for easier excretion by conjugating oestrogen to glucuronide. This is the Phase 2 liver detoxification. Thus, good liver function is necessary for hormone metabolism.

Many people tell me that their GP had ordered a

liver function test (LFT), and it was OK. So why am I so concerned that the liver may not be functioning adequately? For one thing, an LFT does not test liver function. In reality, it is a liver damage test. An abnormal LFT result shows damage. A normal LFT does not necessarily indicate normal/optimal liver function. A better test is a functional liver detox profile (FLDP), which is a test where test substances are given, followed by saliva and urine tests, the results of which show how the body deals with these test substances. This is a more functional test of liver performance.

Good liver function is needed, not just because of hormonal issues, but because we live in a polluted environment. Liver support herbs are important, and I advise all my menopausal patients to use a form of liver support. The most common and probably the best liver herb is St Mary's Thistle.

St Mary's thistle (*Silybum marianum*)

St Mary's thistle, also known as milk thistle, Marian's thistle, holy thistle, and blessed thistle, has been used for liver problems for an extremely long time, going as far back as the ancient Greeks and Romans. Modern research has confirmed what these ancient healers knew; that this herb is very useful for liver problems. St Mary's Thistle can help in healing liver problems, from the serious, such as cirrhosis, viral hepatitis, alcoholic hepatitis, and fatty liver, to the minor and anything in-between. Extracts of this herb have been shown to protect the liver from one of the most hepatotoxic of substances, the death cap mushroom (*Amanita phalloides*) (Abenavoli, Capasso, Milic, & Capasso, 2010).

St Mary's thistle works in three ways.

1) Powerful antioxidants (Silymarin and Silybin, the "active ingredients") in the herb prevent liver damage by preventing free radical damage.
2) It increases the levels of glutathione in the liver, which is probably the most important compound for detoxification of many toxic substances.
3) It stimulates the re-generation of new liver cells.

Liver Support is Essential

The average dose of St Mary's Thistle used in most clinical trials is 140 mg of silymarin three times a day.

The purpose of liver detoxification is to make a substance less active and more soluble to assist in excretion.

Oestrogens can be metabolised down several pathways, but the two major ones are the 2-hydroxy and the 16-hydroxy pathways. The 2-hydroxy oestrogen is less oestrogenic than the original oestrogen, while the 16-hydroxy oestrogen is more oestrogenic.

Therefore, it is important to ensure that the 2-hydroxy pathway is encouraged. This can be done by diet. There are certain compounds in vegetables, especially the cruciferous and mustard vegetables (broccoli, cauliflower, Brussels sprouts, cabbage, kale, kohlrabi, mustard, rutabaga, turnip, wombok and bok choy) that encourage metabolism down the 2-hydroxy pathway.

Indole 3 carbinol (I3C) is a compound found in cruciferous vegetables. I3C encourages metabolism down the 2-hydroxy pathway, thus reducing the concentrations of several metabolites known to activate the oestrogen receptor (Michnovicz, Adlercreutz, & Bradlow, 1997).

I3C works on different levels. Firstly, I3C increases the 2 hydroxylation of oestrogens. Secondly, I3C enhances DNA repair and thirdly, I3C induces gastrointestinal cell cycle arrest and apoptosis. All three activities lead to anticancer effects (Rogan, 2006; Auborn et al., 2003).

Note that I3C is a pro-nutrient. I3C is broken down to di-indolyl methane (DIM) in the stomach and it is the DIM that has the beneficial action on the liver.

I3C and DIM can be supplemented. Some ask if wouldn't it be better to eat the whole vegetable? The problem is that you must eat a lot of broccoli to get the same amount as one capsule of DIM. That is not practical. So, if there is an urgent need to influence oestrogen metabolism, then a DIM supplement can be used. However, a diet high in these vegetables is advisable for ongoing general health.

The recommended dosage of I3C is from 400 to 800 mgs daily. However, Reed et al. (2005) showed that the maximum benefit was seen at a dose of 400mg daily, with no increase found at 800mg daily.

DIM is more stable the I3C and is already the active compound, so smaller doses are needed. The recommended dose of DIM is 100-200mgs per day for women, and 200-400mgs per day for men.

The oestrogens are conjugated, mainly to glucuronide. This makes it soluble enough to be excreted into the bowel via the bile. As in other situations, for this reaction to work adequately, optimal liver function is needed, and this is another good reason for St Mary's thistle to be supplemented.

Other liver herbs include dandelion (*Taraxacum officinale*) and turmeric (*Curcumin longa*).

Gut issues

The oestrogen-glucuronide conjugate is excreted from the liver via bile into the gut. This is not the end of the story. Many things can happen to the oestrogen-glucuronide conjugate before it is finally expelled into the toilet bowl.

Firstly, the longer things stay in the gut, the more likely they will be re-absorbed. So, bowel function is important.

Studies have shown that gut transit time influences serum oestradiol. A faster gut transit time reduces the opportunity to reabsorb oestrogen (Lewis, Heaton, Oakey, & McGarrigle, 1997; Lewis, Oakey, & Heaton, 1998).

Constipation is certainly a factor in the excretion of oestrogen. The more frequently a person has constipation, the more difficult it is to excrete oestrogen. Oestrogen sensitive conditions, such as breast cancer, fibrocystic breast disease, and fibroids, are aggravated by constipation.

Maruti, Lampe, Potter, Ready, and White (2008) concluded that their study *"adds limited support to the hypothesis that increased bowel motility lowers breast cancer risk."*

The converse is that slow bowel motility, i.e. constipation, may well increase the risk of breast cancer. This is because of the increased re-absorption of oestrogen from the gut.

However, the system is not that simple. We know that constipation is more common in pregnancy and menopause.

Women complain of constipation according to their cycle. This suggests that sex hormones may have a role to play in gut motility. Sex hormone receptors have been found in gut smooth muscle (Chen et al., 2019).

Oestrogen can cause constipation (Hogan, Kennelly, Collins, Baird, & Winter, 2009).

So, to regulate bowel function, the diet is very important. The diet must be high in fibre, preferably vegetable fibre, not necessarily grain fibre. Therefore, to avoid constipation, a diet must contain plenty of vegetables, salads, nuts, seeds, and fruit. It is also essential to drink adequate amounts of water. This is part of a good diet, anyway.

There are bacteria in the gut that have a particular liking for glucuronide; and these bacteria release an enzyme called *beta-glucuronidase,* which breaks the oestrogen-glucuronide bond. Once the bond is broken, the bacteria use the glucuronide, and this leaves free oestrogen in the gut. The oestrogen can be re-absorbed/recycled; the extent to which this occurs, as we have seen, depends on bowel transit times. Constipation slows down the transit time, which gives more time for the free oestrogen to be re-absorbed.

The typical western diet, which is highly refined, therefore very low in fibre, predisposes to constipation.

To reduce oestrogen re-absorption, good bowel function needs to be promoted.

Another question to ask is: *"How can we protect the oestrogen-glucuronide bonds?"*

This problem can be approached in two ways: first, the action of the enzyme can be blocked, and second, the number of "bad" bacteria can be reduced.

Calcium D-glucarate

Calcium D-glucarate (also known as calcium D-saccharate) is the calcium salt of the dicarboxylic sugar acid D-glucaric acid. This is a natural substance found in fruits and vegetables, especially oranges, apples, Brussels sprouts, broccoli, cabbage, and bean sprouts. This substance can inhibit *beta-glucuronidase*.

The body eliminates oestrogen and other toxic chemicals by conjugating that substance to glucuronic acid in the liver and excreting it through the bile. *Beta-glucuronidase* can undo this conjugation, which liberates the oestrogen or other toxic chemical into the gut and then it can be re-absorbed rather than excreted. Calcium D-glucarate inhibits this enzyme therefore preventing the de-conjugation and, thus, allows the conjugate to be excreted.

What this signifies is that if there is a high *beta-glucuronidase* level, then oestrogen is not excreted and can be resorbed back into the body. This aggravates the oestrogen dominance and increases the risk of hormone imbalance and hormone dependant cancers.

De-conjugation can be prevented, or reduced, and thus allow the oestrogen to be excreted, simply by eating more of the fruits and vegetables already mentioned or by taking a supplement.

Note some of the better liver detox formulae contain calcium D-glucarate.

Another way to stop or reduce the activity of the *beta glucuronidase* producing bacteria is to supplement with probiotics. By supplementing with "good" bacteria, the "bad" bacteria can be displaced.

Supplement Probiotics

All women being treated for hormonal problems should be encouraged to develop good bowel habits as well as supplementing with 1) a liver support herb, notably St Mary's thistle and 2) probiotics.

Pollution

We have already discussed xenoestrogens: chemical pollutants that have oestrogenic properties, sometimes known as "gender benders". This is because these molecules either stimulate or block the hormone receptors. Consider that for a moment, and you will see the enormity of the problem. Much of our growth and development depends on the right hormone coupling with the right receptor at the right time, and if this beautifully orchestrated process is interfered with, then anything can happen. You don't have to be a rocket scientist to see that the health of the human race is declining. There are more and more cancers, infertility problems, birth defects, sex abnormalities, intellectual problems, mental disease, and so on, and most are because of some hormone interruption.

Almost every product we use has some form of chemical contained within that has some hormone disrupting property. If it doesn't have an effect on hormones, it has an effect on the enzymes.

We are talking about everyday products: personal hygiene products, such as shampoos (average 15 chemicals), perfumes (average 250 chemicals), moisturising creams (average 32 chemicals), lipstick (average 33 chemicals), foundation (average 24 chemicals), eye shadow (average 26 chemicals), nail varnish (average 31 chemicals), deodorant (average 15 chemicals), fake tans (average 22 chemicals), as well as soaps, toothpastes, sunscreens, and so many other products that we use daily.

Chemicals used in plastics, such as bisphenol A (BPA), polyvinyl chloride (PVC), polyvinyl acetate (PVA), polytetrafluoroethylene (PTFE = Teflon®), polychlorinated biphenyls (PCB) and phthalates are also xenoestrogens.

Also, who can forget dichloro-diphenyltrichloroethane (DDT)? DDT is not used now but the residues still remain in the environment.

We all use these products, or they are in our environment, and they have a very negative effect on our health. The levels may not be high, but only small amounts are needed. Also, we have the issue of these chemicals combining to produce synergistic effects. One may be safe, but in combination with two, three, four - we genuinely do not know. What about 500? We definitely do not know!

"Results presented here and elsewhere demonstrate that in combination, chemicals can give oestrogenic responses at lower concentrations, which suggests that in the breast, low doses of many compounds could sum up to give a significant oestrogenic stimulus" (Darbre & Charles, 2010). (Emphasis the author.)

In a study by the Environmental Working Group (EWG), teenagers were screened, and 16 chemicals from four family groups (phthalates, triclosan, parabens and musks) were found in girls aged 15-19 years. These chemicals can be linked to potential health effects, including cancer and hormone disruption. These chemicals are widely found in cosmetics. Every girl tested positive for two parabens: methylparaben and propylparaben.

(https://www.ewg.org/research/teen-girls-body-burden-hormone-altering-cosmetics-chemicals Accessed 2 May 2024)

In an article in the Adelaide *Sunday Mail*, 24 Jan 2010, page 37, research has shown that the average woman applies over 500 different chemicals to her body every day.

In women, especially teenagers, cosmetics can be very dangerous. Perfume, containing up to 250 different chemicals, seems to be the worst. The most concerning fact is that the doses do not need to be high.

Teenagers are in that part of life where the body begins to develop, and the hormones need to work properly to achieve optimal growth and development. One major effect of these chemicals is as a hormone disruptor. What is the result of teenagers using cosmetics that contain these "gender bending" chemicals?

The rate of endometriosis has been increasing over the last 20 - 30 years and is getting worse.

Why?

Could it be due to endocrine disrupting chemicals (EDCs)?

Dutta, Banu, and Arosh (2023) looked at four

endocrine disruptors, *"... (i) polychlorinated biphenyls (PCBs) (ii) dioxins (TCDD) (iii) bisphenol A (BPA) and its analogs and (iv) phthalates ..."*

The researchers concluded that *"The available information strongly indicates that environmental exposure to EDCs such as PCBs, dioxins, BPA, and phthalates individually or collectively contribute to the pathophysiology of endometriosis."*

Hassan et al. (2024) wrote that *"EDCs have been identified to have a deteriorating effect on the female reproductive system, as evidenced by the increasing number of reproductive disorders such as endometriosis, uterine fibroids, polycystic ovary syndrome, premature ovarian failure, menstrual irregularity, menarche, and infertility."*

Endocrine disruptors have been shown to affect or cause,

- the female reproductive system including, in-fertility, early puberty, and early reproductive senescence,
- abnormalities in male reproductive organs,
- reduction in male fertility and reduction in number of males born,
- increase in cancers of breast, ovary, and prostate, and

- increase in obesity and diabetes.

(https://www.niehs.nih.gov/sites/default/files/health/ma terials/endocrine_disruptors_508.pdf Accessed 2 May 2024)

The whole subject of hormone disruptors is very concerning. I would suggest that you read the book 'Our Stolen Future' by Theo Colborn, Dianne Dumanoski and John Peterson Myers.

This may be a little off topic, but to achieve hormonal health, these chemicals must be avoided at all costs. This is difficult, unless you want to live in a bubble, but note that the plastic the bubble is made of may contain chemicals you are trying to avoid. We can minimize their influence by avoiding the products altogether, although this may be difficult. There are personal care products that are chemical free, "natural" or at least contain minimal amounts of chemicals. Use these products. If you have hormonal issues of any sort, avoid chemical laden products as much as possible.

Other forms of chemicals and hormones are in the food we eat. To avoid these, use free range, organic or products specifically labelled "hormone, steroid and antibiotic free".

There are other chemicals that can act as

aromatase up-regulators, meaning that they can increase the activity of the enzyme *aromatase,* which therefore increases the conversion of testosterone to oestrogen (Chen, 2002; Williams & Darbre, 2019).

Examples of the *aromatase* up-regulators are called phenolic endocrine-disrupting compounds (phenolic EDC) such as alkylphenol, chlorinated phenol, bisphenol A (BPA), trichlorsan, octylphenol (OP), nonylphenol (NP). DES can also be added to this list.

The above chemicals may produce more oestrogen, which is not surely a good move, especially if you are a man, or if you are a woman recovering from an oestrogen dependant cancer e.g. breast cancer.

One of the predisposing causes of breast cancer is too much oestrogen; the last thing you want to do is to increase your oestrogen even more.

It is ironic that many women who, after cancer treatment are feeling low, are encouraged to go to the beautician and have a "makeover". This is not necessarily a good thing, as this would include the application of multiple chemicals that are xenoestrogens or *aromatase* up-regulators to their bodies.

Magnesium

Many nutrients are needed and are useful for good health and I have discussed this earlier in this book, and in my other books. I will focus on only one here: magnesium (Mg). As we go on, you will see why it is so important.

First, Mg is usually deficient, especially in Australian society, mainly because Australian soils are lacking in many minerals. It doesn't matter how much broccoli you eat; if the mineral isn't in the soils, it's not in the broccoli!

Second, many in western societies have metabolic syndrome (MetS), where the underlying hyperinsulinaemia (too much insulin in the blood), causes problems. Mg is an intracellular mineral, and insulin is needed to push Mg into the cells. But you may say, if there is more insulin, doesn't this push more Mg into the cells?

No.

Why?

Initially, there may be more Mg pushed into the cells. However, when insulin resistance develops, the body does not listen to insulin and therefore less Mg enters the cells and is lost; urinated out through the kidneys. This leads to Mg deficiency, which, as we have seen, can interfere with the sex hormone biochemical pathways. Mg is also very important in many of the energy pathways, and therefore, a Mg deficiency can lead to poor energy levels. The more common symptoms of low Mg are leg cramps and spasms. Another important symptom is the inability to relax and an inability to fall asleep because the body is tense, and the mind cannot switch off. The common description is that the brain is thinking, thinking, thinking, and cannot switch off! Stress and high cortisol can be another reason for not being able to switch off the brain.

What has Mg to do with menopause? We have already seen that Mg is a co-factor for many enzyme systems, especially in hormone manufacture. Perhaps we should take a step back and have a look at the steroid/oestrogen receptor. Until recently there was only one class of known oestrogen receptor, an intracellular, cytoplasmic receptor, which initiates signal transduction and leads to changes in gene expression over a period of hours to days, i.e. a *slow* process. When oestrogen binds to the receptor, the hormone-receptor complex migrates to the nucleus and binds to a receptor on a section of DNA which then makes new proteins which results in changes in cell function. This process does not need Mg.

However, a new class of oestrogen receptor has been found, a *rapid* acting response signalling membrane receptor. These receptors are a G protein-coupled receptor (Prossnitz et al., 2008).

"G proteins, also known as guanine nucleotide-binding proteins, are a family of proteins that act as molecular switches inside cells, and are involved in transmitting signals from a variety of stimuli outside a cell to its interior."

(https://en.wikipedia.org/wiki/G_protein Accessed 2 May 2024)

Basically, G proteins are an "on-off" switch.

So what?

G proteins *need* Mg to work (Lebbink et al., 2010).

So, we have the situation where,

1) Mg is low,
2) G protein oestrogen receptors need Mg to work optimally, and
3) Oestrogen levels are declining.

So, logically, shouldn't we supplement Mg to try to encourage the body to make more oestrogen by supporting the sex hormone pathways, as well as making the receptor work better, rather than giving oestrogen?

Dose of Mg; a good rule of thumb is to give a maximum of 6 mg per kilogram per day.

Supplement magnesium.

In addition to the diet and life-style changes already mentioned, a triad of

1) Liver support,

2) Probiotics and

3) Magnesium

should be advised.

Herbs

Herbs have been used for a very long time to treat a wide variety of conditions. Herbs were the first medicines before synthetic drugs were introduced. They are not single compounds, but are a mixture of many substances, that have a co-ordinated effect on the body and together add up to a system of checks and balances with a wide window of safety.

In contrast, modern synthetic medicine uses one ingredient, which causes side effects, and the window of safety is very narrow. If a single drug is used, then often another drug in needed to treat one side effect and perhaps more drugs for a third and a fourth and perhaps even a fifth side effect. Herbs have all these checks and balances built into one.

The mistake modern medicine makes is to:

1) discover the "active ingredient" in a herb,
2) isolate it,
3) synthesize it, perhaps even modify it slightly so it can be patented, and
4) push that one component as a drug.

As this process removes all the checks and balances, the final product cannot be as good as the herb.

An interesting question: did women have hormonal issues in the past, or is it only a modern phenomenon? As there is a rich history of herbs used for "women's issues," women in the past must have had problems, although I suspect they were not as common or as severe as today. Many herbs have been used for a very long time to treat menopause and other women's problems.

I will only mention a few as I do not intend to turn this into a herb book.

Maca (Lepidium peruvianum Chacon)

Maca is a root vegetable grown high in the Andes of South America. There are a few species distributed, but only the Lepidium peruvianum Chacon is backed by scientific research (Meissner, Reich-Bilinska, Mscisz, & Kedzia, 2006).

Maca has been used for centuries, both as a food and as a medicine. Folklore has attributed many properties to this plant, which is only now being confirmed by modern research. The plant is similar to a turnip or a radish: it is the root part that is utilised. It contains many vitamins, minerals, alkaloids, tannins and saponins. Maca apparently contains no phytoestrogens and its action on the body is to stimulate the pituitary gland to get the rest of the endocrine glands working again, and it is a natural vitamin and mineral source.

The uses for Maca are many, for both men and women and include menopausal problems, PMT in women, fertility, and erectile problems in men and for energy and stamina in both sexes.

Dong quai (Angelica sinensis)

Dong quai (当归) is a Chinese herb that has therapeutic effects on the female system. It has been used for thousands of years in Traditional Chinese Medicine (TCM), usually in combination with other herbs. In TCM, dong quai is used as a "blood tonic" to nourish the liver and spleen meridians, which influence hormonal balance.

Westerners use this herb in an inappropriate way, according to TCM. That is why it may not always give benefit. TCM use of this herb is for a specific pattern of symptoms. Western use is for a broader "hormonal" use, and in the cases where the herb produces benefit, this may be by chance that it fits into the pattern that is recognised in TCM.

The herb can be useful in PMT (also called PMS in the USA), hot flushes, and any other menstrual, or hormone irregularity. Modern research has shown that the herb produces a balancing effect on oestrogen activity. It is considered an all-purpose women's herb.

Chaste tree berry (Vitex agnus-castus)

This herb was known to the ancients as a treatment

for many gynaecological conditions. Hippocrates (460-370 BC) wrote of this herb "*If blood flows from the womb, let the woman drink dark wine in which the leaves of the Vitex have been seeped*".

Vitex is probably the closest herb there is to progesterone. It does not contain progesterone, but it decreases oestrogen effects and increases progesterone effects by influencing the pituitary gland. It decreases FSH and increases LH, which enhances corpus luteum function. The overall effect is a balancing of the two main hormones.

The herb may be used for PMT, menopausal symptoms and irregular peri-menopausal bleeding.

Black cohosh (Cimicifuga recemosa)

This herb, also known as squaw root, rattle snakeroot and black snakeroot, is a component of the popular menopausal herbal preparation called Remifemin ®. (By mentioning this particular product, I am not endorsing it, nor not-endorsing it.)

It has been used by the Native Americans for female problems for a very long time. Some studies showed that the herb was effective for improving menopausal symptoms, including hot flushes. Not surprisingly, other studies have shown no improvement (Liske, 1998; Osmers et al., 2005).

There has been controversy over the use of this herb. There have been reports of severe liver damage (Whiting, Clouston, & Kerlin, 2002).

The Australian Therapeutic Goods Administration (TGA) looked at 47 cases of liver reactions worldwide (including nine in Australia): at least two in Australia required liver transplantation.

Considering the large number of people taking the herb, the overall incidence of liver reactions is very low. The association is not strictly clear, as other medications were taken concurrently. It is interesting to note that Remifemin ® has been in use since the 1940s in Germany and the reports of liver issues are more recent and very rare.

Are other factors involved, such as other chemicals and drugs in the environment? We do know that one compound may be relatively safe, but when combined with another and another and another, they can act synergistically and become more dangerous. Perhaps the liver cannot cope with all these compounds. Perhaps the herb is the final straw?

This is another good reason to take extra liver support.

A segment on the **7.30 Report** on the ABC on 24 Feb 2010 looked at this herb, especially from the view of dangers. One woman was interviewed who took this herb and developed liver damage, eventually needing a liver transplant. Most of the programme was devoted to the dangers of herbs. There was very little about the fact that the pharmaceutical drugs are dangerous as well, even more so than any herb. The herbalist who was interviewed made the comment that the herb is safe and that there are very rare idiosyncratic reactions. This is what possibly happened in this case.

In the final scene, the woman who had the liver transplant made the comment that the herb was sold in the supermarket, "next to the paracetamol" on the shelves! By saying this, I assume that she implied that the herb is as safe as paracetamol! Most people regard paracetamol (acetaminophen in the USA) as very safe, but the ironic thing is that paracetamol is a potent liver toxin, more so that this herb. Paracetamol is the most common agent in the world causing acute liver failure. In England and Wales, 41,200 cases occurred between 1989 to 1990: this resulted in 150-200 deaths (mortality 0.4%), and 15-20 liver transplants each year (Buckley & Eddleston, 2005)

Between November 2000 and October 2004, the Centres for Disease Control and Prevention, found that paracetamol was the cause of 41% of all cases in adults and 25% of cases in children of acute liver failure (Bower, Johns, Margolis, Williams, & Bell, 2007).

Technically, it is not the paracetamol itself that causes the liver toxicity but a metabolite of paracetamol; N-acetyl-p-benzoquinone imine (NAPQI).

Fenugreek (Trigonella foenum-graecum)

Fenugreek is another herb that can have a beneficial effect on women's health. Note, as will be discussed later, that this herb can also be used for men's health. Fenugreek has been used for centuries in traditional medicine, as attested by references in Ayurvedic and Traditional Chinese Medicine texts.

"... clinical research have outlined the pharmaceutical uses of fenugreek as antidiabetic, antihyperlipidemic, antiobesity, anticancer, anti-inflammatory, antioxidant, antifungal, antibacterial, galactogogue and for miscellaneous pharmacological effects, including improving women's health" (Nagulapalli Venkata, Swaroop, Bagchi, & Bishayee, 2017).

Fenugreek is useful in stimulating breast milk in breastfeeding mothers (Khan, Wu, & Dolzhenko, 2018).

A fenugreek extract has also been shown as *"a useful treatment for increasing sexual arousal and desire in women"* (Rao, Steels, Beccaria, Inder, & Vitetta, 2015).

Kargozar, Azizi, and Salari (2017) researched many herbs and found that fenugreek has positive effects on menopausal symptoms.

As in the male, fenugreek has been shown to be beneficial in diabetes and dyslipidaemia. *"In conclusion, fenugreek improves overall glycemic control parameters and lipid profile safely"* (Kim, Noh, Kim, Choi, & Kim, 2023).

Bio-identical hormones

By the time I see many women with menopausal issues, they have already been to the local health food shop and tried many nutrients and herbs. Others may have been to their naturopaths and have tried the same. Obviously, they do not come to me because they are better: they come to me because they are *not* better. This does not mean that we completely give up on nutrients and herbs, and I recommend that they take St Mary's thistle, probiotics, and magnesium.

Methods of supplementing B-HRT

There are many ways of supplementing B-HRT, but the two most common forms are transdermally as a cream to be rubbed into the skin, or as a troche, which is like a lozenge. The lozenge is not sucked, however, but is allowed to dissolve either under the tongue or between the gums and the cheek so that the hormone is absorbed through the buccal mucosa. The disadvantage is that although some is absorbed through the cheeks, a significant amount is still swallowed.

The issue of the "first pass effect" comes into play when B-HRT is prescribed to be taken this way. This is also the reason hormones are generally not recommended to be given orally as capsules or tablets. Any hormone taken orally is absorbed through the stomach and goes directly to the liver, where a significant proportion is metabolised. To compensate for this, a larger oral dose needs to be given to get the correct dose for the body.

For example, an average dose of transdermal progesterone is 30 mg. This is supplied as a 3% cream (30 mg per gram) To get an equivalent amount by troche, 300mg of progesterone must be given; ten times as much. This would place extra stress on the liver.

B-HRT can also be given as pessaries vaginally, or as suppositories rectally. Both these forms are not very popular, for obvious reasons.

Consent

This is an important issue.

You must ascertain what the person coming to you wants and find out how *they* want to be treated.

Some may answer: *"How should I know? You're the doctor!"* Others may know exactly what they want. They have talked with their girlfriends, their naturopath, or their chiropractor. They probably have not talked with their gynaecologist because gynaecologists are very negative to B-HRT. For them, its synthetic hormones or its nothing. This is strange. As we have seen earlier, the synthetic hormones, especially progestin, have been shown to cause most of the adverse effects. Gynaecologists worry about natural hormones, which have been shown to be safer yet have no issues giving a progestin, which we have seen is more dangerous.

In these modern times, women are very well informed, having researched many sources: books, magazines and the 'net'. Many times, they come with reams of papers showing the latest research. I do not mind this. In fact, I prefer it. You can always learn something new! These women are taking some responsibility for themselves. They are being part of the solution and not part of the problem.

I know many of my colleagues do not like this.

The most important thing is to ascertain that they do not want conventional HRT and are more interested in natural B-HRT. This should be recorded in your notes.

When women are asking for B-HRT, the consent is implied.

Some doctors even request that the women sign a consent form.

Use of B-HRT is still controversial, at least among the mainstream. As we have seen previously, the evidence is that B-HRT is much safer.

Back to the patient.

Where do we start?

The first thing to do is to take a good history. This means, among other things, finding out what symptoms the patient has. It is not good enough to diagnose menopause, all individual symptoms the patient is experiencing need to be recorded. This may be useful in review; you can go through all the individual symptoms and assess improvement.

I vividly remember one lady who came back after six weeks and said she was not much better. So, I referred to my list of her initial symptoms and went through them with her; she was amazed at how many of her symptoms had actually improved. She had forgotten how bad she was originally.

At the first visit, I order tests, and I also discuss the need for dietary change and the use of some supplements, such as magnesium, probiotics, and St Mary's thistle (as discussed above). I may or may not give any B-HRT until the subsequent visit when the results are back. However, if the symptoms are extreme or they have tried herbs, nutrients, diet without success, usually start them on a 3% progesterone cream immediately and still review in four to six weeks' time.

Then, on review, I assess the situation according to the results of the tests, blood or saliva, as well as the response to the diet, nutrients and the progesterone cream. From this, I determine what the next step should be.

Obviously, if they are better with just the nutrients, then we continue and watch and wait.

If they are better with the supplements and the progesterone, I continue with a script for progesterone. I usually start with 3% cream, that is 30 mg of progesterone in 1 gram of cream. I order a 50-gram container which will last for 50 days (just over 7 weeks.) I ask her to return in six to seven weeks.

In the past, B-HRT was supplied in containers that had a nipple on the top. A 1-ml syringe was supplied, which was inserted into the nipple and 1-ml of cream drawn up. This 1- ml of cream was then squirted onto the skin and rubbed in. A newer way of supplying the cream is with a pump pack, which can pump 0.5 ml or 1 ml of cream. For the best results, the site of the cream application should be rotated. The cream and the hormone are fat soluble, so if the cream is applied to the same spot every day, the fat cells become saturated and do not absorb the cream as well. You can apply the cream anywhere you like; but to make a regular habit of using the cream. I suggest the cream is applied to the following areas: 1) left forearm 2) left upper arm, 3) left breast, 4) neck, 5) right breast, 6) right upper arm, 7) right forearm.

My reasoning for this is that there are seven sites and seven days in the week. Once you have reached the right forearm, the cycle can be started again beginning on the left forearm.

This method is generally fool proof, but there have been a few examples where the lady returned after six weeks and said she really was no better. After talking to her, I realized the problem, when she said that she had plenty of cream left. This did not make sense, as I knew I last saw her over six weeks ago and at a dose of 1-ml a day, the 50 ml container should be almost empty. She was using only 0.1 of a ml, not 1-ml of cream. The problem was sorted out by showing her how much cream to apply. On review, after using the correct amount, she was feeling very much better. With the new pump packs, this no longer happens!

The disadvantage of the pump pack is that the amount cannot be varied. Sure, 1 pump, or 2 pumps can be achieved, but not a half pump, three quarters of a pump or one and a half pumps.

With the syringe method, half ml, three-quarter ml, or a quarter ml, can be used as needed.

By now, the results of the blood and/or saliva tests are back, and the formula can be fine-tuned if necessary. Other hormones can be added to the mixture, including oestrogens, testosterone, and DHEA. This is based on individual needs.

Oestrogens come in two forms called biest and triest.

Biest is a mixture of two oestrogens: oestriol 80% and oestradiol 20%.

Triest is a mixture of three oestrogens: oestriol 80%, oestrone 10% and oestradiol 10%.

Biest is generally suggested for the older age group and triest for the younger age group.

Oestrogen deficiency or oestrogen dominance?

Before I go any further, I will address a confusing issue. There is one school of thought that considers women in menopause to be oestrogen deficient and treat it by supplementing oestrogen.

There is another school of thought that says that the main issue is not specifically an oestrogen deficiency, but a progesterone deficiency.

As women age, the level of oestrogen declines, and menopausal symptoms develop. When these women are tested, a low oestrogen level is found; a low level as compared to a younger woman.

So, yes, these women have an oestrogen deficiency. You can see how easy it is to consider the problem as primarily an oestrogen deficiency. Going back to the time of Dr Robert Wilson and his book, 'Feminine Forever,' menopause was regarded as solely an oestrogen deficiency, so from the beginning, all the symptoms of menopause were regarded as part of an oestrogen deficiency.

This is interesting as some symptoms such as moodiness, breast soreness and swelling, and heavy periods are actually symptoms of excess oestrogen. How can we have symptoms of excess oestrogen when there is an oestrogen deficiency?

Nature is not always that straight-forward.

We should realize that hormones do not travel alone: they usually occur in pairs. One hormone having an antagonistic effect on the other. The car accelerator and brake scenario. We should not look at oestrogen on its own. We should look at oestrogen (the accelerator) in context with progesterone (the brake). Oestrogen is the accelerator; it makes things grow.

Why are those males who wish to become women prescribed oestrogen? To make breasts grow.

Why do elderly men grow "man boobs" ("moobs")? This happens because the relatively excess oestrogen caused by *aromatase,* converts testosterone to oestrogen.

Why do women with anovulatory cycles have heavier periods? This occurs because oestrogen makes the uterine lining thicker and there is no progesterone to modify this.

As women age, oestrogen declines (oestrogen deficiency). However, progesterone also declines, although much more so than oestrogen; so, we have an oestrogen deficiency, but also an even greater reduction of the braking effect of progesterone, so we have a *relative* excess of oestrogen compared to progesterone. This is the oestrogen dominance that I made mention of earlier.

There are other reasons for a relative excess oestrogen,

1) Xenoestrogenic pollutants,
2) Chemicals in personal care products, and
3) The inability of the body, especially the liver, to excrete oestrogen.

We discussed these earlier.

In summary, there may be an *absolute* oestrogen deficiency but a *relative* oestrogen excess, which is out of proportion to the progesterone.

To deal with this problem, the oestrogen/progesterone ratio needs to be balanced by supplementing progesterone.

This idea of oestrogen dominance and progesterone deficiency was promoted by Dr John Lee, whose book 'What Your Doctor May Not Tell You About Menopause' has already been mentioned.

So, which is it? Low oestrogen or low progesterone? You could say that this goes to the heart of the matter; women should be assessed individually, based on their symptoms and on their hormone profile that can only be determined by doing appropriate tests. Then, and only then, can we be sure that we can supplement the correct hormones.

Each script for hormone replacement is a therapeutic trial; the formula given is based on history, examination, and investigations. After each review, the formula may be changed (fine-tuned), until it is correct, and the patient is satisfied with the results.

Each woman is an individual and therefore should be treated on an individualised basis. The same goes for men and the same goes for the treatment of any other non-sex hormone issue.

Women going through menopause present with a number of symptoms. To refresh your memory of these, refer to the symptoms listed earlier.

Doctors practicing alternative medicine break up the symptoms as below:

Oestrogen deficiency: hot flushes, night sweats, vaginal dryness.

Progesterone deficiency: moodiness, irritability, teariness, anxiety, depression, loss of confidence, poor memory, lack of concentration, headaches, "cotton wool head", palpitations, insomnia or sleep disturbances, muscle/joint aches and pains, dry skin, and hair.

Mainstream doctors would say all the symptoms are due to oestrogen deficiency.

Who is right?

The adage, 'the proof of the pudding is in the eating,' comes to mind.

Which women feel better? The ones on oestrogen or the ones on progesterone? Of course, some may need both.

However, in over 30 years of experience prescribing B-HRT, with progesterone as the main hormone being replaced, I can say that the progesterone deficiency is the dominant picture.

Of course, I cannot give a "set in concrete" protocol of hormones because each woman is an individual and needs individual treatments. This is one of the other primary advantages of compounded B-HRT; it allows for individualised formulae for each woman.

Some women do very well with progesterone only replacement. However, there are some women who need oestrogen replacement as well.

I reiterate a warning mentioned earlier; women should not be replaced with oestrogen alone. If oestrogen needs replacing, then it should be together with progesterone (the accelerator and the brake).

A good question to ask is "Why can we give progesterone alone but not oestrogen?" This is related to the fact that first, the dominant pattern is one of progesterone deficiency and second, our environment is full of xenoestrogenic pollutants. So even if the blood test shows a low endogenous oestrogen level, that person's body is probably full of other oestrogens from the pollution. Progesterone needs to be given to overcome the effects of these oestrogen mimickers or blockers; "gender benders". The pollutants are oestrogenic, not progestogenic.

321

Some women do need oestrogen replacement, especially for intractable hot flushes or vaginal dryness. However, as mentioned above, this needs to be supplemented in conjunction with progesterone.

Some women may need progesterone, oestrogen, DHEA, and testosterone. To find the right formula and dose is a matter of testing and then trial and error.

If there is a regular cycle, and there would be in the younger woman, then the use of hormones must follow the physiological cycle. By this I mean that if progesterone is being supplemented, then it must be used physiologically. Generally, the menstrual cycle is 28 days. Day 1 is defined as the first day of menstrual bleeding, day 14 is the day of ovulation and day 28 is the last day of the cycle, just as the bleeding starts: day 28 of the cycle is the same as day 1 of the next cycle. Generally, in the first half of the menstrual cycle, progesterone levels are low and at about day 14, with ovulation, progesterone levels rise. Note that the follicle that ovulates forms the *corpus luteum*, which secretes the progesterone. Also note, if there is no ovulation, there is no *corpus luteum* and, therefore, no progesterone. The life span of the *corpus luteum* is two weeks, so after two weeks the *corpus luteum* fails, the level of progesterone drops, and this helps to initiate the next period.

Physiological replacement refers to both amount and timing. Therefore, the correct amount of progesterone must be supplemented at the correct time: from day 14 (ovulation) to day 28 (start of period). In summary, this means two weeks off (day 1-14) and two weeks on (days 14-28).

In menopausal women, the cream can be used continuously. The problem comes with women who have irregular cycles. Here we can either use the cream cyclically or use continuously, depending on the age or other factors. The period can be regulated by using the cream two weeks on, two weeks off. The cream can be stopped if a period starts, then stop for two weeks, then start again. By doing this, the period can be regulated to a 28-day cycle.

In some cases, the woman may feel good while on the cream but feels unwell on days 1-14 when she is not using the cream. Progesterone can be used throughout the cycle, but in a physiological manner.

Here, a specific case comes to mind. The lady in question felt great from day 14 to 28 but absolutely awful from days 1-14, so I suggested she take a small dose from days 1-14, then a larger dose, then increase further in a step-up fashion and then reduce closer to day 28. With trial and error, she worked out that she needed ¼ ml cream from days 1-10, then ½ ml from days 11-14, then 1 ml from days 15-26, then ¾ ml from day 27 until her period.

This mimics the hormonal rises and falls more accurately. Luckily, this method is only required for the exceptional cases. This takes some trial and error. In this case, the woman was part of the solution; one who was willing to experiment with herself a bit.

There are times when finding the correct dose can be difficult. One way to deal with this situation is to give a prescription of progesterone and biest in separate containers. This allows the woman to trial varying doses of the two different creams, adjusting the doses by trial and error until the optimum formula is found, saving both time and money, since the person does not have to keep returning to the surgery to have the doctor make the changes.

This may not work for everyone, but it is especially good for the enthusiastic, "switched on" woman who wants to be part of the solution.

The myth of hysterectomy

According to mainstream thought, once a woman has had a hysterectomy, she no longer needs to use progesterone. They seem to think that progesterone receptors only exist in the uterus. Mainstream doctors use mainly progestins such as medroxyprogesterone acetate (MPA) and MPA only works on progesterone receptors in the uterus, therefore it is correct to say that if there is no uterus, then there is no need for progestogens! However, as we have seen earlier on, progesterone receptors *do* exist in many other tissues. "Real" progesterone needs to be used, hysterectomy or not, to influence progesterone receptors all over the body.

Women who have had a total hysterectomy, i.e. womb and ovaries removed, need all hormones supplemented, which could include progesterone and oestrogen, as well as DHEA and testosterone. So here we can get creative. The formula you design needs to fit the woman. This can be determined by saliva testing, by symptoms and by how well she feels.

For example, a typical formula is progesterone 3%, testosterone 1%. Occasionally, oestrogen needs to be added. Generally, only a small amount is needed, for example, biest 0.2%, although sometimes a higher dose is needed.

DHEA 1-2% can also be added if there is stress, adrenal issues, or tiredness and the DHEA levels are low.

This formula does not need to be "set in concrete". At each review, depending on symptoms, and depending on test results, the formula can be fine-tuned. Ongoing review and monitoring are necessary.

Pregnenolone

DHEA is often referred to as the "mother of all hormones". If that is so, then pregnenolone could well be called the "grandmother of all hormones."

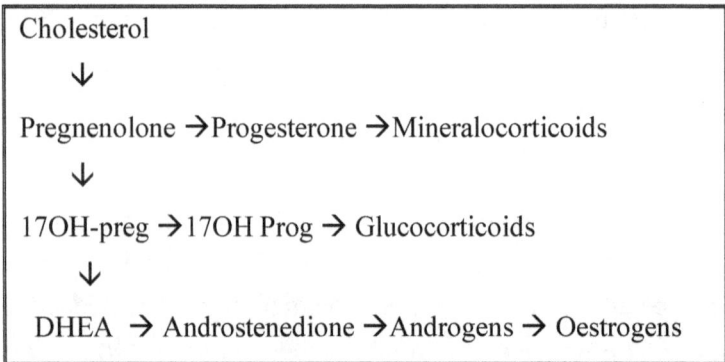

Cholesterol

↓

Pregnenolone →Progesterone →Mineralocorticoids

↓

17OH-preg →17OH Prog → Glucocorticoids

↓

DHEA → Androstenedione →Androgens → Oestrogens

Pregnenolone is the precursor of *all* the steroid hormones. The first step in steroid production is the conversion of cholesterol to pregnenolone, which is then converted to all the other steroids. See diagram.

A valid question to ask would be: Why not supplement the one "grandmother" hormone to make all the others rather than supplanting all the end hormones?

While there is some logic to this, unfortunately, it is not so simple. For pregnenolone to be converted to the other hormones, enzymes and co-factors are needed. As discussed earlier, this is dependent on the nutritional status of the individual, and we know that the level of nutrition is generally poor.

Also, the level and activity of these enzymes decrease with ageing. Meldrum, Davidson, Tataryn, and Judd (1981) showed that pregnenolone levels do *not* decline with age, while other hormones, notably DHEA, do decline with age. The researchers concluded that the decline in hormone was due to an age-related change in enzyme activity, rather than a decline in pregnenolone *per se*.

However, there is a contrary opinion that claims pregnenolone levels *do* decline with age and this is used to promote pregnenolone replacement. Animal experiments show a decline in brain levels of pregnenolone, and this is related to a decline in cognitive function (Mayo, Le Moal, & Abrous, 2001; Vallée et al., 1997).

As mentioned before, the issue of whether results in animal studies can be extrapolated to humans remains undecided.

Pregnenolone receptors are found in the brain. This suggests that pregnenolone is a "neuro-steroid" which means it must have some action on brain function. Studies have shown lower levels of pregnenolone in those with schizophrenia (Ritsner, Maayan, Gibel, & Weizman, (2007), in patients with generalized social phobia (Heydari, & Le Mellédo, 2002), depression (George et al., 1994), and Alzheimer's disease (Weill-Engerer et al., 2002).

Pregnenolone has been found to have other actions including reducing allergic reactions, as a memory enhancer, fatigue reliever, stress reducer, antidepressant, anti-inflammatory for rheumatoid arthritis, prevention of dementia and as a nerve regenerator.

Dosage of pregnenolone

Pregnenolone is quite safe and can be supplemented in a cream or a troche. The general principle, as with other hormones, is to start low, using, for example, 10 mg and slowly titrate upwards. Monitoring is usually done by measuring pregnenolone levels, but if this test is not available, oestrogen, testosterone, progesterone, and DHEA levels can be measured.

These measurements, as well as the response of the patient, will help the practitioner to achieve an optimal dose. A generally accepted maximum is 100mg per day, although as there is little research, this is not a fixed, determined maximum dose. Note, however, that these are relatively conservative doses because in the 1940s and 1950s, much higher doses were used. In a review published by Henderson, Weinberg, and Wright, (1950) pregnenolone was shown to be safe, even in high doses.

Studies in the 1940s showed that pregnenolone can be used in the treatment of rheumatoid arthritis in doses up to 300mgs per day without any major side effects (Myers, 1951).

Side effects are generally related to overdosage. Excess doses can cause irritability, anger, anxiety, insomnia, acne, hair loss (excess conversion to androgens), headaches, heart irregularity and palpitations. I repeat, the side effects are related to an excessive dosage. Therefore, it is wise to start with a low dose and slowly increase, as clinically indicated.

Side effects

Is B-HRT safe?

Or should the question be: - "Is B-HRT safer than other hormone replacements?"

The question of safety and side effects of B-HRT has been answered already. The answer is a conditional "yes" and my reasons for this is explained in this book.

B-HRT consists of molecules that are structurally the same as those made by the body, therefore, in themselves they cannot be considered dangerous. This should be compared with "new to nature molecules" where we are not always sure what their effects are. This is *physiology* versus *pharmacology*.

Another issue is related to the amount supplemented.

Too little will not achieve the required level and, therefore, will not produce optimal beneficial effects. Too much will produce the side effects of excess hormone.

I have heard the comment from some people that they had tried B-HRT, and it did not work. Perhaps we should re-phrase that statement; B-HRT did not work for them, at *that* dose, *that* length of time used, or *that* formula.

The difficulty is getting the right dose and the right proportion of hormones. Trial and error with monitoring and review and fine tuning can achieve the correct dose for each individual person.

Many times, in this book, I have referred to physiological replacement. This means giving a dose that produces normal physiological levels, which have the desired positive effect without over-dosing to produce symptoms of excess, hence the need for regular monitoring and review.

Giving a natural molecule at a physiological level cannot possibly be dangerous.

Another reason for side effects is not the hormone *per se*, but the vehicle the hormone comes in, that is, the substances the cream or the troche is made from. In the last thirty years, I can count on one hand the number of people who had a reaction to the vehicle. Compounding pharmacists generally use a low allergenic base, although we know that some people can be allergic to almost anything. Different creams or bases can be utilized in the rare cases where there is an unwanted reaction.

Progesterone and neuroprotection

I have already looked at the neuro-protective function of progesterone. Progesterone protects the brain from trauma. Is this why women tend to recover better from brain trauma or strokes than men?

Why would nature make progesterone neuro-protective?

Let's consider what happens at childbirth. In natural childbirth, a baby is pushed out, headfirst usually through a narrow opening. What can this do to the baby's brain? Squeeze it and squash it. Do babies' brains recover from this trauma? More often than not: yes.

Could the high level of progesterone in the mother's body during the end of pregnancy be acting on, protecting and saving the baby's brain?

It makes sense. Nature has provided a mechanism to protect the baby from the trauma of birth by producing a high progesterone level in the mother.

The placenta makes huge amounts of progesterone as well as other neuro-protective steroids, which have a role in protecting the foetal brain (Hirst, Palliser, Yates, Yawno, & Walker, 2008).

There is enough research to support giving a progesterone supplement to anyone who has sustained brain trauma, a stroke, or any other form of brain injury, whether male or female. Progesterone protects the brain and helps it to heal.

Progesterone and anti-ageing

Earlier I mentioned the branch of medicine known as "anti-ageing medicine". I mention this again because there is some evidence to show that supplementing hormones has an anti-ageing effect. Topical progesterone has been used as an anti-ageing and skin firming treatment for some time. Progesterone cream has been sold in the USA as an "over the counter" moisturising cream for years.

Holzer, Riegler, Hönigsmann, Farokhnia, and Schmidt (2005) investigated the use of a 2% progesterone cream in a double-blind randomised, vehicle-controlled study. Skin elasticity, epidermal hydration and skin surface lipids, clinical monitoring, self-determination as well as blood tests (LH, FSH, oestrogen and progesterone) were studied.

"The results of this study demonstrate that topical 2% progesterone acts primarily in increasing elasticity

333

and firmness in the skin of peri- and postmenopausal women. These effects, in combination with good tolerability, make progesterone a possible treatment agent for slowing down the ageing process of female skin after onset of the menopause."

In another study, synthetic hormones, norethisterone acetate and ethinylestradiol were used orally. These synthetic hormones did *not* improve the skin, indicating that there is a difference between the natural and the synthetic.

"Low-dose hormone therapy for 48 weeks in postmenopausal women did not significantly alter mild to moderate age-related facial skin changes" (Phillips, Symons, Menon; HT Study Group., 2008).

If you are thinking it is because the first study was transdermal and the second study was oral treatment, an earlier study looked at both.

Twenty-four women were assigned to three therapy groups, as well as a placebo group.

1) Transdermal oestrogen only
2) Transdermal oestrogen and 0.4 mg progester-one vaginal pessary
3) Oral oestrogen and 0.4mgs progesterone vaginal pessary
4) Control group

Here we are comparing oral oestrogen vs transdermal oestrogen and transdermal (vaginal) progesterone vs oral oestrogen and transdermal (vaginal) progesterone. The end result was that all three regimes significantly improved parameters of skin ageing (Sator, Schmidt, Sator, Huber, & Hönigsmann, 2001).

The big difference with the quoted study was that a synthetic progestin was used.

As mentioned before, there is a difference between the natural and the synthetic. Natural is definitely better.

Where do you get it?

B-HRT is generally available only from compounding pharmacists. These are specialist pharmacies where the pharmacist goes back to basics and mixes these compounds to make the creams and troches on their premises. They do not just type out a label and stick it onto a box or bottle as other pharmacists do.

The compounding pharmacist makes up the cream or the troche according to the formula given by the prescribing doctor. This indicates that the prescribing doctor must be familiar with, and be knowledgeable about, making up these formulae.

There are some doctors who have not studied the topic yet still think they can prescribe B-HRT. They and their patients are the ones that may get into difficulties because of inappropriate formulae.

Conventional prescribing does not need much thinking as medications are generally standardised to only a few strengths.

The doctor who writes out the script for B-HRT can inform you where the nearest compounding pharmacist is, or you can find one on the internet.

Conversely, you can contact your nearest compounding pharmacist to find a doctor near you who is familiar with B-HRT.

ANDROPAUSE

Men also go through a form of menopause, although it may not be recognised as such. Andropause, the male equivalent of menopause, can be a much more subtle event. Many of the symptoms are non-specific and often considered a part of ageing.

This may be part of the problem.

How can you differentiate andropause from "just ageing"?

Is it the same thing?

In the woman, the lead up to menopause, and the final cessation of menses, is characterised by widely fluctuating changes in periods that can be dramatic and very noticeable. Women's hormones tend to fluctuate more, which can lead to emotional and physical changes that become issues for the woman, as discussed in the previous chapter.

All through life, men's hormones are more stable, and the slow decline may be missed. Men do not have periods and sometimes it is difficult to tell if there is anything wrong. However, even if they do not notice them, men have changes. A part of the problem for men is that even if they notice changes, they do not generally like to complain, or they become embarrassed and tend not to speak out about what they are experiencing.

The changes may be slow, and many men do not notice certain changes, such as personality transformations, where they become more emotional, more moody, more grumpy. It is the people around them, especially their spouses and work colleagues, who may notice something is going on.

Men experiencing hormonal changes may notice that they are losing strength and perhaps motivation. One thing that they definitely do notice, and which is possibly the worst thing that could happen, is the loss of erections. This is something that cannot be missed, and many men become depressed because of this loss and are too embarrassed to seek help.

To most men, the erection is the sign of manhood; and so, when unable to have an erection, men are not men. Because of this, they may become depressed and may also go through a "mid-life crisis", where they evaluate their lives and decide that they have achieved little.

Some men state that they don't know why they are depressed. Although as you read through this chapter, it maybe you notice the purported unknown reason is often not so much unknown as deliberately unacknowledged.

Other men may do the opposite. Their "mid-life" crisis consists of trying to prove that they are *not* having problems. They buy a brand-new sports car and have an affair with their 25-year-old secretary!

"Scientists have found a way to keep middle-aged female mice from going through menopause. Now they're working on a way to keep middle-aged male mice from buying expensive sports cars."

Conan O'Brien (1963-) American television host, comedian, writer, and producer.

When men have problems and refuse to discuss them, they develop into "grumpy old men"!

How can we, as practitioners, help them?

First, we must recognise that there is a problem.

For too long, it was not accepted that men would experience hormonal changes. If the problem is not recognised, then there is no problem! This is not fair to the men.

So, what is this problem that causes distress in men?

With women, the problem is a reduction in hormones, as discussed in the previous chapter. In men the problem may also be a hormone reduction, and that hormone is testosterone.

Testosterone is generally referred to as the "male hormone", although women also have it and may need supplements. Men also have oestrogen and progesterone, the "female hormones", however in different proportions.

A large portion of "maleness" depends on testosterone. A deficiency of this hormone causes a loss of "maleness", and this is the cause of many of the emotional and psychological problems men have as they grow older.

Some more confident, self-assured men do not worry; they just accept this as a part of "natural ageing".

Symptoms of andropause

Before we can diagnose a condition, we have to know what the symptoms are. The top six symptoms of andropause are:

1) Depression
2) Sweating and hot flushes
3) Decreased libido and erectile dysfunction
4) Fatigue
5) Poor concentration and memory
6) Loss of motivation

Other symptoms include decreased muscle mass, sleep disturbances, osteoporosis, body fat gain, especially abdominal, aches and pains, and loss of height. Many of these symptoms are subtle, non-specific and may be considered a diagnosis in their own right.

For example, if an elderly man becomes depressed, he is diagnosed with depression and put on an anti-depressant.

Depression is *not* a disease; it is a symptom of an underlying problem. So, do we diagnose "depression" and treat with an anti-depressant, or do we look for a reason and treat the underlying cause? This man may be going through andropause, and depression is one of many symptoms. It would be more appropriate to treat the andropause-caused depression with testosterone replacement, rather than anti-depressant medication, which will not get to the root cause for the depression.

Testosterone testing

As a part of a full assessment of any male, testosterone levels need to be measured. In the previous chapter, I discussed hormone measurement using either blood or saliva testing, and which is more effective. The same applies here. To recap, saliva testing measures the "free" hormone, in this case testosterone. Blood tests show the total testosterone, but the binding proteins need to be measured to calculate the "free" testosterone.

As discussed earlier, the saliva testosterone test is not covered by Medicare, and many cannot afford this test. The next best thing is a blood test.

A serum testosterone is relatively useless on its own. As explained earlier, hormones do not float freely in the blood and only the "free" hormone is biologically active. There are carrier proteins that bind a large proportion of the testosterone, and it is very important to know the level of SHBG and albumin, as this can give us an idea of the "free" testosterone, which is the biologically active hormone.

When you are ordering blood tests, it is essential to request "Androgen Studies". This test includes:

1) Total testosterone,
2) SHBG,
3) Albumin, and
4) Calculated free androgen index (FAI), or "free testosterone".

If levels of testosterone are low, then this can be correlated to the symptoms described by the person.

Automatically prescribing testosterone replacement is not necessarily the first choice.

Before even considering the use of testosterone replacement, things like diet, nutrients, herbs and supplements must be considered. Men seeking help are often of the same philosophy that was discussed with women's hormones.

Some men have done their research and want to go on to testosterone immediately.

Also, many have already been to the health food shop and have tried the various herbs and nutrients that are on the market. There is a great deal of hype and powerful advertising with these herbs and many men try them. Of course, if men try them and find they make a difference, then they do not need to go to the doctor!

343

A valid question to ask is: *"How effective are these herbs that are advertised for men's problems?"*

There are many herbs used for men's potency, so these issues must have been a problem in the past. It is not a recent phenomenon.

Herbs: the science and the hype

Sex sells!

Anything that increases sexual performance sells.

Before the days of the "little blue pill" there was virtually nothing else on the market.

Because sex is so important to most men, and because having an erection is a sign of manhood for many, most men would be prepared to do almost anything that might help.

In the 1920s and 1930s men went to the extreme of having surgeons transplant monkey testes tissue (monkey glands) on to their testes. The surgeons who did so, did it for "therapeutic purposes"! (Dr Serge Voronoff (1866-1951) was the main proponent.)

Some heavily advertised herbs have been described as being "scientifically validated" to help the drooping male appendage and male libido. However, the quality of some of that research is questionable.

A search of the internet finds many sites trying to sell these herbs. The advertising points to some research, yet the source of the research is rarely mentioned.

Despite this, many men have tried these products, and, anecdotally, they do help some, but not all. This can be said about any product; herbal or pharmaceutical!

These herbs have been used for centuries for much the same reason we are using them today. We know they are safe; the experience of herbalists for centuries can attest to this.

Are they effective? As, they have been used for centuries, they must work, otherwise they would have ended up in the dustbin of useless remedies long ago!

Tribulus terestris

One of these herbs is *Tribulus terestris*. Tribulus has been used for centuries in Traditional Chinese Medicine (TCM) and Ayurvedic Medicine. The herb has many properties, having an effect on digestion, as an expectorant, a demulcent, a diuretic, a liver tonic, a stamina enhancer and as an aphrodisiac. It has mainly been promoted for the last two purposes.

There is some confirmatory science, but then there is also a lot of hype. Companies began to manufacture products containing this herb (plus others) and the products were heavily promoted. Remember, at this time there was nothing much else available. Men bought these products, and they became very popular.

BUT *"Do they work?"*

Tribulus terestris, also known as *puncturevine, caltrop, cathead, yellowvine, goathead* and *bai ji li* (Chinese 白蒺藜) is an herb that is reputed to increase testosterone levels in men with subsequent increase in strength, muscle bulk and sexual performance.

You can see why this herb became popular.

Some studies had come from the Soviet Bloc, mostly from the Chemical Pharmaceutical Research Institute in Sofia, Bulgaria in the 1970s, showing that Tribulus increased testosterone levels by increasing luteinizing hormone (LH) levels. Elevated LH stimulates the testes to make more testosterone. This study from Bulgaria has been quoted, quoted again and re-quoted, however the original study seems to have been lost, as I could not find it!

The herbs became popular for the treatment of sexual disorders as early as 1981 in the Soviet Bloc, which then filtered through to the west.

A more recent study that is accessible has shown that Tribulus does not influence androgen production in young men (Neychev & Mitev, 2005).

However, animal studies have shown increased levels of testosterone. In a recent study, Tribulus was given to primates, rabbits and rats (including castrated rats). The active chemical in Tribulus terrestris is protodioscin (PTN). The active compounds are called steroidal saponins.

"TT (Tribulus terestris) increases some of the sex hormones, possibly due to the presence of protodioscin in the extract. TT may be useful in mild-to-moderate cases of ED. (Erectile dysfunction)" (Gauthaman & Ganesan, 2008).

In another study, also using animals, *"These results were statistically significant. It is concluded that TT extract appears to possess aphrodisiac activity, probably due to androgen increasing property of TT (observed in our earlier study on primates)"* (Gauthaman, Adaikan, & Prasad, 2002).

Note: These studies were done in animals, and it seems that the herb does have an effect on animals.

"But what effect does it have on human males?"

Unfortunately, there are only a few small studies available. Some studies looked only at performance enhancing effects of the herb and unfortunately, the results were not positive. So, in these studies, the science negated the hype.

Rogerson et al. (2007) studied twenty-two elite male rugby players who were randomly given Tribulus or placebo. The researchers concluded that *"T. terrestris did not produce the large gains in strength or lean muscle mass that many manufacturers claim can be experienced within 5-28 days. Furthermore, T. terrestris did not alter the urinary T/E ratio and would not place an athlete at risk of testing positive based on the World Anti-Doping Agency's urinary T/E ratio limit of 4:1."*

Antonio, Uelmen, Rodriguez, and Earnest (2000) studied the effect of Tribulus on fifteen resistance-trained males. The group was randomly assigned to Tribulus or placebo. The researchers concluded that *"Supplementation with tribulus does not enhance body composition or exercise performance in resistance-trained males."*

Does Tribulus have a real effect on men's hormonal systems and/or libido and sexual function? There are studies that show it does not, but some studies do show a positive effect.

Gamal El Din et al. (2019) concluded that *"... this study replicates the findings of previous reports about the robust effect of this herbal medicine (Tribulus) in elevating the testosterone level and improving the sexual function of patients who suffered from erectile dysfunction with partial androgen deficiency.*

Of course, there are many anecdotes about the usefulness of Tribulus.

Despite this, the herb must have some action. After all, many men do take the herb and are satisfied with the results (or is it a placebo?). I repeat: if this herb did *not* work, then the use of it would have died out years ago.

Some assert that Tribulus does not increase testosterone to a supra-physiological level. Nor does it appear to do much in men with normal levels, however, it may benefit men with low levels of testosterone.

Horny goat weed

Horny goat weed (*Epimedium grandiflorum,*

Epimedium brevicornum) is reputed to have aphrodisiac properties. According to legend, a Chinese goat herder noticed increased sexual activity in his flock after eating this plant, hence the name!

The active ingredient in this herb is *icariin,* and this substance is supposed to increase levels of nitric oxide (NO), as well as inhibiting the enzyme *phosphodiesterase type 5* (PDE-5). PDE-5 is the enzyme that is responsible for degrading cGMP, which is created by NO. Sildenafil, the "little blue pill" is also a PDE-5 inhibitor. By blocking this enzyme, the breakdown of NO is reduced, so it has a longer effect, thus producing an erection.

Dell'Agli et al. (2008) were studying herbal extracts to look for a compound similar to sildenafil. They found one component of horny goat weed, *icariin,* to have PDE-5 inhibiting effects. They then modified icariin, to make it much more potent. The researchers suggested that this compound was *"a promising candidate for further development."*

There is a study performed by Dr Steven Lamm MD and Gerald Secor Couzens who compared a group of men taking a proprietary combination of *Epimedium grandifloris*, *maca, mucuna pruriens* and *polypodium vulgare* with a group of men taking sildenafil.

They concluded that *"Daily use of the herbal complex for a minimum of 45 days resulted in an enhancement of sexual satisfaction in 60 percent of healthy male subjects and 45 percent of men using Viagra. The exact mechanism of action of the herbal mixture is unknown although it may have a testosterone-like effect."*

This is another study that is quoted and re-quoted on many websites selling horny goat weed, yet there is no mention where the paper was published - if it was published at all. I could not find the original study.

Horny goat weed, also known as *yin yang huo (*淫羊藿) has been used in Traditional Chinese Medicine (TCM) for a very long time. TCM considers this herb as a kidney yang tonic, though it is almost never used alone. Westerners buy this herb on its own and then find it may not work. In the same category, Tribulus, which is known as *bai ji li* (白蒺藜), is also used in mixtures and is not considered to have any sexual stimulating function. TCM uses this herb for liver problems and for wind.

Muira puama

Another herb used in men's hormonal problems is

Muira puama, also spelled mara puama, marapuama, and marapama. Botanically, this herb belongs to the genus *Ptychopetalum* and there are only two species: *Ptychopetalum olacoides* and *Ptychopetalum uncinatum*. For herbal use, the *P. olacoides* is preferred because of the higher content of *lupeol*, one of its main phytochemicals. This herb is also known as potency wood. It is a small Brazilian tree that grows across the Amazon River basin and has a long history of use in Brazilian folk medicine as an aphrodisiac, as well as for fatigue, musculo-skeletal problems and rheumatism.

But, as with others already discussed, *"Does it work?"* There have been a few small studies which showed benefit in poor libido and erectile dysfunction. Proper scientific studies are, however, are currently lacking.

There is one study of a Brazilian herbal formula in women:

"The efficacy of a unique herbal formulation of Muira puama and Ginkgo biloba (Herbal vX) was assessed in 202 healthy women complaining of low sex drive."

The researchers continued, *"Responses to self-assessment questionnaires showed significantly higher average total scores from baseline in 65% of the sample after taking the supplement. Statistically significant improvements occurred in frequency of sexual desires, sexual intercourse, and sexual fantasies, as well as in satisfaction with sex life, intensity of sexual desires, excitement of fantasies, ability to reach orgasm, and intensity of orgasm. Reported compliance and tolerability were good. These initial findings support the strong anecdotal evidence for the benefits of Herbal vX on the female sex drive. A double-blind study is planned to further research these results"* (Waynberg & Brewer, 2000).

One thing we do know…it is safe.

"In Brazil, a herbal medicinal extract named Catuama containing a mixture of Paullinia cupana (guarana; Sapindaceae), Trichilia catigua (catuaba; Meliaceae), Ptychopetalum olacoides (muirapuama; Olacaceae) and Zingiber officinale (ginger; Zingiberaceae) is used as a body stimulant, energetic, tonic and aphrodisiac. The present study investigated the chronic administration of 25 mL Catuama twice a day during 28 days for any toxic effect on healthy human volunteers of both sexes. No severe adverse reactions or haematological and biochemical changes were reported" (Oliveira et al., 2005).

Research on another herbal mixture VigRX, containing Epimedium leaf extract, Cuscuta seed extract, Ginkgo Biloba leaf, Asian Ginseng root, Saw Palmetto berry, Muira Pauma bark extract, Catuaba bark extract, and Hawthorn berry, showed some benefit in premature ejaculation (Raisi, Farnia, Ghanbarian, & Ghafuri, 2010).

Fenugreek

Fenugreek (*Trigonella foenum-graecum*) is another herb that has androgenic and anabolic effects in the male. Mansoori, Hosseini, Zilaee, Hormoznejad, and Fathi (2020) concluded that *"Results from clinical trials suggest that fenugreek extract supplement has an effect on serum total testosterone levels in male."*

Rao, Steels, Inder, Abraham, and Vitetta (2016) showed that a fenugreek extract improves age-related symptoms of androgen decrease, increases testosterone levels and improves sexual function in healthy aging males.

Qiu et al. (2024) showed that fenugreek improves type 2 diabetes (T2D) and its complications by improving diabetic endothelial dysfunction, leading to an increase in nitric oxide (NO) production. Fenugreek also increases testosterone levels which also improves endothelial dysfunction.

This improvement in testosterone levels, improved endothelial function and increased NO production, can improve erectile difficulties.

Tongkat Ali

Tongkat Ali (*Eurycoma longifolia*) is another herb reputed to increase men's potency. This herb has been used traditionally in Southeast Asia as an anti-malarial, anti-pyretic, anti-ulcer, cytotoxic and as an aphrodisiac. Again, this focus on aphrodisiac and sexual enhancer caught the eye of many westerners. Not to say that the local inhabitants haven't used it for the same purpose!

The reputed mode of action is that it increases levels of testosterone. Bodybuilders have used this herb to increase muscle mass. There is some evidence that Tongkat Ali does what it says. Hamzah and Yusof (2003) showed that Tongkat Ali increased muscle strength and size when compared to placebo.

Leitão, Vieira, Pelegrini, da Silva, and Guimarães (2021) concluded that *"The combination of Eurycoma longifolia and concurrent training improved erectile function and increased total testosterone levels in men*

355

with ADAM (androgen deficiency of ageing males)."

A study by Leisegang, Finelli, Sikka, and Panner Selvam (2022) concluded that E. longifolia can be a safe and promising option for hypogonadal men.

There are plenty of animal trials. My favourite title is: **Sexual arousal in sexually sluggish old male rats after oral administration of Eurycoma longifolia Jack** (Ang, Lee, & Kiyoshi, 2004).

You can just imagine a group of scientists in white lab coats with clipboards, looking at old fat rats trying to mate!

The paper states that *"Tongkat Ali.... has been used in Malaysia to increase male virility and sexual prowess."* and *"We conclude that the results of this study support the folk use of this plant as an aphrodisiac."*

In another study, Ang, Ikeda and Gan (2001) concluded that *"These results provide further evidence that E. longifolia increases the aphrodisiac potency activity in treated animals.*

And another.

Effects of Eurycoma longifolia Jack (Tongkat Ali) on the initiation of sexual performance of inexperienced castrated male rats (Ang, Cheang &

Yusof, 2000).

And another: -

Eurycoma longifolia Jack enhances libido in sexually experienced male rats (Ang & Sim 1997).

So, what can we conclude?

There are plenty of animal studies to show that these herbs work. Unfortunately, there is little scientific human data.

There is much anecdotal data, and we also have the knowledge from the traditional use of the herb, which can go back many generations. Herbalists, healers, shamans pass on their knowledge from one generation to the next, so there may be thousands of years of experience with these particular herbs. It may not be consistent with modern scientific procedure, but the knowledge is there. The fact that people have continued to use the herb down through the ages is an indication that they must work. If over time, the herb was obviously not working, the use would have stopped.

It seems that Tongkat Ali can increase testosterone levels in hypogonadal men but does not increase testosterone levels to supraphysiological levels in men with normal testosterone.

Dr Peter Baratosy MBBS FACNEM

As a good summary, Adimoelja (2000) wrote that *"Traditional herbs have been a revolutionary breakthrough in the management of erectile dysfunction and have become known worldwide as an 'instant' treatment. The modern view of the management of erectile dysfunction subscribes to a single etiology, i.e. the mechanism of erection. Many pharmacological agents are orally consumed and vasoactive agents inserted intraurethrally or injected intrapenially to regain good erection. Modern phytochemicals have developed from traditional herbs. Phytochemicals focus their mechanism of healing action to the root cause, i.e. the inability to control the proper function of the whole-body system. Hence phytochemicals manage erectile dysfunction in the frame of sexual dysfunction as a whole entity. Protodioscin is a phytochemical agent derived from Tribulus terrestris L plant, which has been clinically proven to improve sexual desire and enhance erection via the conversion of protodioscine to DHEA (De-Hydro-Epi-Androsterone). Preliminary observations suggest that Tribulus terrestris L grown on different soils does not consistently produce the active component Protodioscin. Further photochemical studies of many other herbal plants are needed to explain the inconsistent results found with other herbal plants, such as in diversities of Ginseng, Eurycoma longifolia, Pimpinella pruacen, Muara puama, Ginkgo biloba, Yohimbe, etc."*

There are very limited human studies. Many of the studies are inconsistent and while some are promising. More research is needed.

"However, the majority of research into the safety and efficacy of medicinal plants or herbs are mainly based on animal models and very limited studies on humans, probably due to negative clinical trial results, drug interactions or toxic reactions" (Low & Tan, 2007).

Srivatsav et al. (2020) writes, that *"While L-arginine is a safe supplement with clinical data supporting improved erectile function, limited data exist on the efficacy of other ingredients in the treatment of ED."*

L-arginine will be discussed later.

Herbs are like grapes. The quality of wine made from the grapes depends on the soil, the climate, whether grown on the "sunny side of the hill", the amount of water, time of harvest, and so on. Herbs grown in different soils can have different properties, so it is important to standardize herbal products to avoid any variations.

It is possible that many studies on humans will not be done because herbs cannot be patented. What drug companies do is to isolate the "active ingredient", make a modified form and then patented that. Only then will drug companies become interested because such a process means they will make money! However, that is not herbal medicine; it is a modified "active ingredient" with all the checks and balances removed and which in the long run may cause more side effects.

What other supplements can be used in andropause?

I have made mention of one of the major features of andropause, and that is erectile dysfunction (ED).

How can we treat this problem, other than with the "little blue pill"? We have seen some evidence that the above-mentioned herbs may help.

Is there a specific nutrient that can also help?

Yes.

If we look at the physiology of erections, we see that one of the main molecules needed is nitric oxide (NO). The enzyme, *PDE-5* is also implicated as it breaks down the NO. So, we can either inhibit the *PDE-5* or make more NO. We have seen that the horny goat weed has a *PDE-5* inhibiting effect.

How can we increase NO?

Can we supplement NO?

We cannot because it is a gas, but we can supplement the precursor of NO.

L-arginine

The amino acid, L-arginine, is the precursor of NO, which is involved in achieving erections. L-arginine if found naturally in meats, eggs, dairy, nuts, and seeds, in fact, in any good protein source.

L-arginine can also be given as a supplement.

NO is a powerful vasodilator and is not only useful in ED but also in hypertension.

One of the issues with L-arginine is that it needs to be taken regularly, unlike the "little blue pill" which can be taken on an "as needed basis". One study has shown that, if needed, a large dose of L-arginine can be used "as needed".

Does L-arginine work?

There have been studies that have shown success.

In one study, Stanislavov and Nikolova (2003) gave L-arginine to 40 men in combination with

Pycnogenol, which is known to increase NO by stimulating *nitric oxide synthetase,* the enzyme that converts L-arginine to NO. On the equivalent dosage of 1.7 gm of L-arginine and Pycnogenol 40 mg tablets three times a day, there was significant improvement.

Note: Pycnogenol is a proprietary brand of pine bark extract that contains proanthocyanidins, a polymer of flavonoids, which are powerful antioxidants. They can also be found in grape seed extract, cinnamon, cocoa, apples, red wine, green tea and other similar foods.

"We conclude that oral administration of L-arginine in combination with Pycnogenol causes a significant improvement in sexual function in men with ED without any side effects."

In another study, Lebret, Hervé, Gorny, Worcel, and Botto (2002) gave a 6-gram dose of L-arginine with yohimbine hydrochloride 6 mgs one to two hours before intended intercourse. Yohimbine is a herb from Africa that also has sex boosting properties.

I purposefully do not discuss yohimbine further as it is not legal in Australia.

"This pilot study shows that the on-demand oral administration of the L-arginine glutamate 6g and 6 mg yohimbine combination is effective in improving erectile

function in patients with mild to moderate ED. It appears to be a promising addition to first-line therapy for ED."

When L-arginine was given alone at a dose of 500mg three times a day, the conclusion was that *"Oral L-arginine 3 x 500 mg/day is not better than placebo as a first-line treatment for mixed-type impotence"* (Klotz, Mathers, Braun, Bloch, & Engelmann, 1999).

Is it that the L-arginine alone does not work, or does it mean the dosage given was too low?

Chen et al. (1999) used a much higher dose, 5 gm per day.

"Oral administration of L-arginine in high doses seems to cause significant subjective improvement in sexual function in men with organic ED only if they have decreased NO excretion or production. The haemodynamics of the corpus cavernosum were not affected by oral L-arginine at the dosage used."

Dosage: from the above studies, we can conclude that L-arginine 500mg on its own is inadequate. 1.7 gm in combination with Pycnogenol 40 mgs three times a day does work. A 5g dose daily does work. So, either you give a high dose alone, or give a lower dose in combination with another herb or antioxidant.

Something to be considered in this discussion is a relationship between erectile dysfunction (ED) and cardiovascular disease. The state of the arteries is essential for achieving an erection. To put it bluntly, if the arteries in the penis are working, then the arteries in the rest of the body should also be working. Conversely, if there is ED, then we can assume that the penile arteries are not working and therefore the arteries in the rest of the body are damaged.

Erectile function is a sensitive indicator of cardiovascular health and can be used as a marker for pre-morbid heart disease (Billups, Bank, Padma-Nathan, Katz, & Williams, 2005).

Basically, if you do not have any issues with ED, then your heart health is probably good as well.

What is the point of saying what I just did?

The use of the "little blue pill" to "treat" ED is only symptomatic and temporary. There is no long-term artery benefit. On the other hand, the regular use of L-arginine will have long-term protection and therefore benefit arterial function.

There is a related PDE-5 inhibiting drug called tadalafil. While sildenafil has a short length of action (two to four hours), tadalafil's length of action is up to thirty-six hours. A low dose of 5 mg daily can be used long-term. It not only has beneficial effects in achieving erections on demand but can also have positive effects on benign prostatic hypertrophy (BPH) (Mónica & De Nucci, 2019), and pulmonary hypertension (Galiè et al., 2009). It also has cardiovascular protective effects, for example in coronary heart disease, hypertension, heart failure, and pulmonary arterial hypertension as well as in diabetes mellitus (Liu, 2013) due to its vasodilating effects.

Dealing with the underlying issues is more important.

In one of the studies quoted above, the use of L-arginine with Pycnogenol showed great improvement in ED. This is because:

1) L-arginine is the precursor of nitric oxide (NO).
2) Pycnogenol has been shown to stimulate *nitric oxide synthetase,* the enzyme that converts l-arginine to NO.

If, at the same time, a PDE-5 inhibitor is used, such as horny goat weed, then the rate of NO metabolism is reduced. Smooth muscle relaxants keep arteries open. NO is the molecule that is the most important of these.

We can go one step further. *Nitric oxide synthetase* is produced in the endothelial cells and is dependent on the endothelial cells working optimally. As we have seen, endothelial dysfunction is one of the earliest problems in MetS. The state of the arteries is paramount. If we can save our artery lining, the endothelium, we can prevent heart disease and ED. As noted above, fenugreek has been shown to have endothelial protecting properties.

How do we protect our arterial lining?

Diet is obviously an important factor. We can start off by recommending the low stress diet (LSD). This diet is high in antioxidants and protein. Protein is a good source of L-arginine. Perhaps the most important benefit is that it is low in sugar, is known to be complicit in causing endothelial dysfunction.

A highly refined carbohydrate diet can lead to hyperinsulinaemia, which we have seen does have an effect on hormones. A low protein diet can lead to increased levels of SHBG with a resultant decrease in "free" testosterone (Longcope, Feldman, McKinlay, & Araujo, 2000).

So, to protect the endothelium, we need to keep testosterone levels up, therefore a higher protein diet should be followed.

Other advice includes losing weight, (which is part of the LSD), stop smoking, reduce alcohol and to exercise more and improve fitness levels.

Many men, especially the elderly, have a poor diet, one that is especially low in protein.

So, as the adage goes: *"Feed the man meat!"*.

It is very important to keep "free" testosterone levels up in males. Even if we cannot increase testosterone (without supplementation) we can advise a diet that can decrease SHBG, which can increase "free" testosterone. We know that sugar not only decreases SHBG but also is unhealthy. In the long run, sugar causes more health problems and should be avoided.

For many years, the myth has been that testosterone *causes* heart disease. This is now known to be false. In fact, low testosterone levels can cause heart disease and probably other vascular disease.

It is important to keep testosterone levels up in men.

"In conclusion, a low plasma testosterone level was associated with endothelial dysfunction in men independent of other risk factors, suggesting a protective effect of endogenous testosterone on the endothelium" (Akishita et al., 2007).

So, to protect the endothelium, testosterone levels need to be optimised.

Exercise

Exercise is very important. Not only does it help with weight loss, but it also helps to improve muscle strength as well as mood. A fitter male feels better and performs better at work and in the bedroom!

Exercise can increase testosterone levels (Schwab, Johnson, Housh, Kinder, & Weir, 1993).

Exercise can prevent ED, and where ED has already begun, exercise can improve this (Derby et al., 2000).

The type of exercise you do is important! Bicycle riding may make ED worse, due to the bicycle seat pressing onto the perineum.

"Straddling bicycle saddles with a nose extension is associated with suprasystolic perineal compression pressures, temporarily occluding penile perfusion and potentially inducing endothelial injury and vasculogenic ED" (Huang, Munarriz, & Goldstein, 2005).

There are many factors to consider when choosing this kind of exercise, including hours of cycling, the weight of the cyclist, the skill of the cyclist and, most importantly, the fit of the bicycle, especially the fit of the bicycle seat. Specially designed seats can reduce this problem.

Sex can also be considered as exercise (sexercise?). However, many older men worry that they may die while having sex. This is an unfounded fear. *"Middle-aged men should be heartened to know that frequent sexual intercourse is not likely to result in a substantial increase in risk of strokes, and that some protection from fatal coronary events may be an added bonus"* (Ebrahim et al., 2002).

On the other hand, Fisher et al. (2012) showed that there seems to be an increased incidence of cardiovascular events in men having an extramarital affair.

Why?

We can speculate that perhaps it would be due to the extra stress or guilt. I will let the readers think about that one!

Vitamin D

Vitamin D has been shown to have many uses, such as for heart protection, for cancer prevention, for boosting immunity, for bone building, among others. Some research has shown a novel effect of Vitamin D.

Vitamin D can be considered a steroid hormone!

As it is made from cholesterol, vitamin D also has a steroidal structure.

Higher vitamin D has been shown to be associated with higher levels of testosterone. There is a concordance between vitamin D levels and testosterone levels. In the summer the levels are higher than in winter. *"Men with sufficient 25(OH) D levels (>/=30 mug/l) had significantly higher levels of testosterone and FAI and significantly lower levels of SHBG when compared to 25(OH)D insufficient (20-29.9 mug/l) and 25(OH)D deficient (<20 mug/l) men (p<0.05 for all)"* (Wehr, Pilz, Boehm, März, & Obermayer-Pietsch, 2010).

Extra sunshine, sun exposure, not sun burn, and/or a vitamin D supplement may be a good idea if testosterone levels need to be increased. However, there are many people who are constantly in the sun Their deeply tanned skin is an obvious indicator. (Beware of the fake tan, though!) However, on testing, many have an unexpectedly low vitamin D (25 hydroxy vitamin D) level.

Why?

Perhaps there is a biochemical block. The conversion of pro-vitamin D to 25 hydroxy vitamin D is a reaction needing magnesium (Mg). We have already seen that the level of Mg is quite low in western societies. Mets, which is very common in western society, is also associated with low Mg levels. These people may need Mg supplementation as well as a vitamin D_3 supplement. The active vitamin D is 1, 25 dihydroxy vitamin D, and this conversion is made in the kidneys and requires zinc.

Why should there be this connection between vitamin D and testosterone? Perhaps it is an evolutionary thing. Could it be related to seasons and sunlight and procreation? Winter can be a good time for making babies! Long cold nights, but nine months later is already autumn and a newborn may not survive as well in the coming cold winter. So, in winter, there may be a lower testosterone, therefore less mating! With a nine-month gestation, mating in spring/summer (high vitamin D, high testosterone) and the baby will be born in the next spring, which may give the best opportunity for survival.

This is just speculation on my part!

Summary

- Eat well
- Eat fewer, or hardly any refined carbohydrates
- Eat more protein
- Stop smoking
- Reduce alcohol

371

- Exercise more
- Have more sex (not extramarital)
- Get more sunshine

Testosterone replacement therapy (TRT)

If a patient has made dietary changes, has tried the various herbs, and is still not feeling well, and/or the testosterone levels are low on either salivary or blood testing, the next step can be to supplement testosterone and/or DHEA, which also has androgenic effects.

Conventional medicine is now also advocating testosterone replacement. Pharmaceutical companies are manufacturing various synthetic testosterone products, although lately they are making more "body-identical" (bio-identical) testosterone products. Remember Schopenhauer.

We have already discussed bio-identical hormones.

Where do we start when considering testosterone replacement?

Of course, it is always a good idea to fully examine the man before starting any hormone. An essential check is for prostate problems. Check especially for prostate problems using both a digital rectal examination (DRE), and a blood test, specifically measuring prostate-specific antigen (PSA). This is for the protection of the practitioner as much as it is for the patient.

We discussed the testosterone-cancer connection in the first half of this book and there is a big question-mark between prostate cancer causation and testosterone.

Despite evidence of testosterone providing a protective factor against cancer, the mainstream still believe that testosterone causes cancer. If soon after you put a put a male onto testosterone, a prostate cancer is diagnosed, it is certain that you, the practitioner who started the patient on testosterone, will be blamed. So, cover yourself. If your preliminary tests pick up a suspicious lump or an elevated PSA, this will have to be investigated before going further.

You are now ready to prescribe testosterone.

You have a male patient in front of you who is complaining of various symptoms. He describes general vague symptoms but some of them such as weakness, loss of motivation, depression, moodiness, and loss of libido, sound familiar. He is in the susceptible age group - over 50, and you immediately suspect andropause. Your response is to check the testosterone levels before doing anything else.

The results come back as low. I then discuss andropause with the patient, and since the testosterone levels are low, I suggest he start to make dietary changes and add nutrients and herbs. Together with the patient, a review in six weeks is planned. When he returns, he says he is not better. I then suggest we can start plan B – testosterone replacement therapy (TRT).

I generally start with a 5% cream (5% = 50 mgs per gram) and suggest a starting dose of 0.5 ml of cream per day to rub into the skin and rotating the sites. This can be increased slowly to 1 ml or more if needed. Of course, there must be follow up and regular monitoring to prevent over-replacement.

For the same reason mentioned above, i.e. the first pass effect, testosterone should not be given orally. The cream form is better, as transdermal hormones bypass the first pass effect.

From here on, it is a matter of trial and error. Check symptoms, assess improvement, examine saliva or blood tests to monitor progress, then modify the dose if necessary.

An average dose in men ranges from 5% (50 mg /day) to 10% (100 mg per day).

As has been discussed, sometimes women may need some testosterone. Doses for women are one tenth lower than those for men: 0.5 mg to 1 mg daily, or 0.5% to 1% cream. Testosterone is generally not used on its own in women, it is mixed in with oestrogen and/or progesterone. Occasionally, testosterone cream 1% can be used separately but concurrently with the progesterone and/or biest cream or troche.

Mainstream medicine uses oestrogen in the treatment of urinary incontinence. This is based on the fact that vaginal oestrogen can be used for an atrophic vaginal mucosa. They extrapolate that if oestrogen can help the vaginal mucosa, then it could help bladder problems; yet the studies show not only that it doesn't work but that it can make thing worse. There is some evidence that testosterone, not oestrogen, can help.

Urinary incontinence can be treated by applying testosterone cream 1% to just inside the vagina.

What else can testosterone cream be used for?

I am told by women who have tried it, who are reliable sources, that applying testosterone cream directly on the clitoris before sex can help anorgasmic women.

In all cases, the underlying principle is to supplement testosterone as a therapeutic trial.

375

If the person improves and has a better quality of life, then continue the same dose with appropriate monitoring (PSA, cholesterol, testosterone levels, and SHBG.).

If there is no improvement, then adjust the dose and continue to monitor symptoms and salivary or blood testosterone levels. If there is still no improvement, you may have to re-assess the person. Look for issues mentioned earlier, e.g. smoking, alcohol, drugs, diet, exercise, for example.

If there is increased moodiness and irritability, consider over-dosage. This is a good reason to monitor the levels.

Low testosterone does not occur in isolation. There may be other diseases present, the most common being MetS but there may be others such as hypothyroidism.

Diet, exercise and supplements such as chromium, zinc, and selenium, are needed. An important point to mention is that testosterone can be used to treat MetS.

"Testosterone replacement therapy improves insulin resistance, glycaemia control, visceral adiposity and hypercholesterolaemia in hypo gonadal men with type 2 diabetes" (Kapoor, Goodwin, Channer, & Jones, 2006).

There may be one danger with testosterone replacement in men. We do not want the testosterone to be converted to oestrogen. In earlier discussion of the enzyme *aromatase,* we saw how in many men, testosterone can be converted to oestrogen. This is clearly evident in older, obese men who frolic on the beach with their large "man boobs" / "moobs". In these men, it is obvious that their testosterone is being converted to oestrogen.

This is not a good thing for males.

Aromatase can be inhibited.

Zinc is an effective *aromatase* inhibitor. A daily dose of 15-30 mgs should be adequate. As already mentioned, the best source of zinc is meat.

Another good reason to *"Feed the man meat!"*

Another *aromatase* inhibitor is chrysin.

Chrysin

Chrysin is a bioflavonoid extracted from the blue passionflower (*Passiflora caerulea*). Chrysin has poor oral bioavailability and therefore must be supplemented via a non-oral route, either transdermally as a cream, or as a troche (Walle, Otake, Brubaker, Walle, & Halushka, 2001).

There are oral preparations of chrysin available. Although earlier studies showed a poor oral absorption, it seems that this is improved if the chrysin is mixed with piperine, an extract from black pepper.

Chrysin has been shown to be a potent *aromatase* inhibitor.

"Chrysin, the most potent of the naturally occurring flavonoids, was similar in potency and effectiveness to AG (aminoglutethimide), a pharmaceutical aromatase inhibitor used clinically in cases of estrogen-dependent carcinoma. These data suggest that flavonoid inhibition of peripheral aromatase activity may contribute to the observed cancer-preventive hormonal effects of plant-based diets" (Campbell & Kurzer, 1993).

Use is generally as a cream ranging in potency from 5 to 20%. This can be added to the testosterone cream. For example, a formula such as testosterone 10%, chrysin 10% to be applied 1 ml cream daily.

One problem with chrysin is that it has a yellowish colour and may stain clothes or bed linen.

Dihydrotestosterone (DHT)

In the first part of the book, DHT was mentioned as an alternative to testosterone replacement, the main reason being that DHT cannot be aromatised. A*romatase* does not convert DHT to oestrogen.

This can be a significant advantage.

We discussed earlier that testosterone can be aromatised to oestrogen and this can have detrimental effects on the prostate. In the discussion, we considered the use of testosterone replacement but then realized that some of this testosterone can be converted to oestrogen. We have looked at ways of preventing this by supplementing aromatase-inhibitors, such as zinc and chrysin.

This may not be necessary if DHT is supplemented instead of testosterone.

However, there is always this worry that DHT, a more androgenic androgen, may be dangerous. There is especially the concern that DHT may cause or aggravate benign prostatic hypertrophy (BPH) or prostate cancer. As explained in the first half of the book, this is not a concern. DHT, on its own, does not cause BPH or prostate cancer. What is more of a concern is the oestrogen caused by the aromatisation of testosterone. If androgens need to be supplemented in andropausal men, why not supplement DHT? There is a definite advantage, as it cannot be aromatised.

Studies have shown that DHT supplementation to elderly men is safe and effective. Effects on the prostate, lipids and other blood parameters are not significant.

Kunelius, Lukkarinen, Hannuksela, Itkonen, and Tapanainen (2002) performed a double-blind study where men were put on varying doses of DHT (125-200mgs per day) and compared to a placebo group. The researchers concluded that *"Transdermal administration of DHT improves sexual function and may be a useful alternative for androgen replacement. As estrogens are thought to play a role in the pathogenesis of prostate hyperplasia, DHT may be beneficial, compared with aromatising androgens in the treatment of ageing men."*

Ly et al. (2001) studied men who were put on 70 mg transdermal DHT gel compared with placebo. The researchers concluded that DHT transdermally is safe, effective and had no adverse effects.

Dosage of DHT ranged from 70mg per day, through to 200mg per day. A good policy is to start low and slowly work up, adjusting the dose to the benefits received.

There is always concern about cancer and heart disease when people are started on testosterone, however I addressed this concern earlier in the book.

As with women's B-HRT, testosterone cream needs a script from a registered medical practitioner, preferably one who is experienced in natural hormone treatment. The prescribed medication must be able to, ideally, be dispensed from your local compounding pharmacy.

Look on the internet for a compounding pharmacist. The doctor prescribing the medication can inform you where the nearest compounding pharmacy is. Conversely, contacting a compounding pharmacist can also inform you where the nearest B-HRT experienced doctor is.

The prostate

The prostate is a walnut sized gland situated in the male pelvis beneath the bladder. The anatomical curiosity is that the urethra, the bladder outlet tube runs through this gland, so it is not hard to see why enlargement of this gland causes urinary problems: the enlarging gland squashes the outlet tube.

The most common form of prostate problem is

benign prostatic hypertrophy (BPH).

The most common symptoms are urinary in nature including,

- poor stream,
- dribbling,
- difficulty in starting or stopping urination,
- feeling that urination has finished–zip up then having a leak and wetting self,
- urgency,
- feeling of not being done,
- increased frequency, especially at night (nocturia). This can vary from 1 to 2 times a night to every 2 hours. This certainly has a negative effect on sleep, and
- discomfort generally but can cause pain.

BPH is also considered inevitable in all males. The incidence increases with age, especially after the age of 40. By age 50, 50% of all men have some degree of BPH. By age 80, the incidence is as high as 80%. However, only 25% of men will need to be treated by age 80.

The mainstream considers that the development of BPH is related to testosterone and DHT, though newer studies put this idea into some doubt. As we have seen in the first half of the book, how can a hormone that is declining cause this? Unless it is the deficiency, that is the cause. This flies completely in the face of mainstream thinking. As we have seen, it is not necessarily the testosterone but the oestrogen that is the major culprit; to be precise, it is the oestrogen/testosterone ratio. An increasing oestrogen and a decreasing testosterone are the problems, especially if *aromatase* is converting all the testosterone to oestrogen!

This does not mean that testosterone and DHT play no part. These androgens act in a permissive role.

As discussed earlier, a declining testosterone, a rising SHBG and a rising oestrogen level are the problems. We have already looked at ways of increasing testosterone and decreasing SHBG and oestrogen.

Firstly, we need to reduce the level of oestrogen. This can be achieved by reducing the conversion of testosterone to oestrogen by the enzyme *aromatase.* The most important *aromatase* inhibitor is zinc. As we have seen above, another inhibitor is chrysin.

Men can also use DIM and/or I3C, and/or calcium D glucarate to reduce oestrogen levels.

We can also increase testosterone by diet and exercise and vitamin D as noted above.

SHBG can be reduced by diet and exercise.

The mainstream way of treating BPH is to try to reduce the formation of DHT by inhibiting the enzyme *5 alpha reductase*. There are drugs that can do this, and the claimed success is about a 30% reduction in prostate size. Of course, if DHT is the sole cause of BPH, this is a fairly poor result. So other factors *must* be involved.

There are herbs that can do the same job with even better results because they work on different levels.

Saw palmetto

Saw palmetto, Latin names: - *Sabal serrulata* or *Serenoa repens*, common names: - American dwarf palm tree and cabbage palm, is a small palm tree native to eastern United States. The berries are the main part of the tree used.

This herb has multiple actions:

1) Sabal has a *5 alpha reductase* inhibiting action (Weisser, Tunn, Behnke, & Krieg, 1996),
2) Sabal inhibits the binding of DHT to prostatic cells (el-Sheikh, Dakkak, & Saddique, 1988), and
3) Sabal inhibits various inflammatory activities

(Breu et al., 1992).

From this, it can be seen that Sabal works at different levels, not just by inhibiting *5 alpha reductase.*

Nettle root extract

Another herb that is very useful in BPH is the common garden nettle *Urtica urens,* and *Urtica dioica,* (both found worldwide), and *Urtica incisa,* which is native to Australia. Nettle is a weed that most people would find annoying in their garden, but it is a very useful herb. The different species are considered therapeutically interchangeable.

Extracts from the root have been shown to influence the prostate, on different levels.

1) There is inhibition of *sodium potassium ATPase,* an enzyme that is essential for cell growth (Hirano, Homma, & Oka, 1994),
2) Nettle root extract inhibits SHBG attaching to its receptor and therefore prevents the SHBG-oestrogen induced amplification of the andro-gen signal (Hryb, Khan, Romas, & Rosner, 1995).

Epilobium

Epilobium species (*Epilobium angustifolium, Epilobium parviflorum and Epilobium hirsutismpiriform*) is another popular herb used in prostate problems. This herb also works on many levels.

1) Epilobium has been shown to inhibit the growth of human prostate cells (Vitalone, Guizzetti, Costa, & Tita, 2003). This growth inhibiting effect was non-specific, inhibiting growth in four different human cell lines (Vitalone, McColl, Thome, Costa, & Tita, 2003).

2) Epilobium has also been shown to have *5 alpha reductase* inhibition activity, as well as *aromatase* inhibition activity (Ducrey, Marston, Göhring, Hartmann, & Hostettmann, 1997).

Proprietary prostate herbal mixtures can contain zinc, Sabal, Epilobium and/or nettle extract, as is evident from the above descriptions, many levels of prostate metabolism can be affected.

Are these herbal mixtures effective? Sökeland (2000) studied a pharmaceutical synthetic *5 alpha reductase* inhibitor and compared it to an herbal mixture (Sabal and Urtica). The result was that the effectiveness was much the same, but the herbal mixture had better tolerability, in that it had fewer side effects.

The long-term efficacy and safety of herbal treatment was assessed as "excellent" (Lopatkin et al., 2005).

Prostate cancer

Many doctors are afraid to give elderly men testosterone replacement because of the fear of cancer.

As discussed earlier, testosterone may not specifically cause prostate cancer; however, it would be prudent to assess each person with the minimal of a digital rectal examination and a serum PSA.

It would be unwise to give testosterone to anyone with overt prostate cancer. However, testosterone replacement does not seem to have any effect on a normal prostate or with cases of sub-clinical prostate cancer.

Prostate cancer can be prevented by encouraging a good diet, especially a diet low in refined carbohydrates, sugar, and so on, and high in protein and "good fats" especially omega-3 fatty acids (fish oil). "Bad fats" such as *trans* fatty acids, or rancid fats, should be avoided.

Cooked tomatoes, which contain lycopene, can also be beneficial. Other sources of lycopene include guavas, watermelon, red capsicum (bell peppers), persimmon, asparagus, red cabbage, and mangos.

Other nutrients that are helpful in preventing prostate cancer include zinc, selenium and plenty of antioxidants such as vitamin C.

Sunshine (vitamin D) is also very important. Vitamin D has been shown to be useful in the prevention and treatment of prostate cancer (Chen & Holick, 2003).

Epilobium has been shown to reduce prostate cell growth (Vitalone, Guizzetti, Costa, & Tita, 2003).

Reduction of obesity is important, and this has a connection with MetS. We have seen that obese men have a higher incidence and a more aggressive prostate cancer than thinner men. Obese men also have more *aromatase,* converting testosterone to oestrogen.

We have already discussed the need to prevent/reduce the conversion of testosterone to oestrogen by inhibiting *aromatase.* Zinc is a good *aromatase* inhibitor (Om & Chung, 1996), hence the need for an adequate zinc intake.

Lycopene

Lycopene is a red-coloured carotene found in tomatoes and other red-coloured fruits and vegetables such as red carrots, watermelons, papaya, pink grapefruit, and others, although it is not found in strawberries or cherries.

This carotene has been known to have a positive effect on the prostate. Lycopene has been shown to inhibit the progression of BPH (Schwarz et al., 2008) and has also been shown to have a beneficial effect on prostate cancer (Kucuk et al., 2002).

A diet high in these red coloured fruits and vegetables will have a favourable effect on prostate problems. A high intake of tomatoes and tomato products is associated with a lower incidence of prostate cancer (Giovannucci, Rimm, Liu, Stampfer, & Willett, 2002).

Therefore, the population of men who eat lots of tomatoes should have lower rates of prostate cancer. In fact, Mediterranean men have a lower mortality rate from prostate cancer compared to northern European men (Kenfield et al., 2014; Giovannucci et al., 1995), which may be due to the higher tomato intake as part of the Mediterranean diet.

The method of preparing tomatoes is relevant. Cooked, processed tomatoes have more bioavailable lycopene that raw tomatoes. Soares et al. (2019) wrote *"Lycopene is more bioavailable in processed tomato products than in raw tomatoes, since arrangement of cis-isomers of lycopene during food processing and storage may increase its biological activity."*

In women, lycopene has been shown to have a beneficial effect on the breast and cervix. Giovannucci (1999) wrote, *"The evidence for a benefit was strongest for cancers of the prostate, lung, and stomach. Data were also suggestive of a benefit for cancers of the pancreas, colon and rectum, esophagus, oral cavity, breast, and cervix."* (Emphasis the author.)

Progesterone

Men also make progesterone, although not as much as women. What little they do make is needed. Progesterone influences the prostate.

If we consider the car accelerator/brake scenario, where oestrogen is the accelerator and progesterone is the brake, then this scenario works in the male as well as the female. Progesterone is known to antagonise the effects of oestrogen. Oestrogen has been shown to be a major factor in the development of prostate hyperplasia as well as cancer, then the use of progesterone in prostate problems makes sense. There is certainly clinical and anecdotal evidence, but is there any scientific proof?

Progesterone also may inhibit prostate cancer growth by inducing apoptosis. We saw earlier that the p53 gene induces apoptosis in breast cancers. This gene is also found in the prostate gland. Progesterone up-regulates this gene to increase apoptosis (programmed cell suicide).

However, when we look at more aggressive prostate cancers, the ones that have metastasised, we find that the p53 gene has mutated. This is perhaps one reason why it has become more aggressive, as there is inactivation of the p53 pathway, although there are other alternative signalling systems as well (Osman et al., 1999).

Since progesterone up-regulates to p53 gene and increases apoptosis in breast cancer, why shouldn't it do the same in prostate cancer?

Studies in the 1950s showed progesterone was beneficial in the treatment of prostate cancer (Trunnel, Duffy, Marshall, Whitmore, & Woodard, (1951); Trunnel, Duffy, Marshall, Whitmore, & Woodard, (1950). Unfortunately, there has been little work done on this recently.

New progesterone derivatives have been

synthesized and have shown positive benefits in experiments with hamsters looking at prostate and prostate cancer (Cabeza et al., 2006).

Another factor known to influence the p53 gene is zinc. Zinc deficiency has been shown to have a negative effect on the p53 gene (Fanzo et al., 2001).

Zinc deficiency reduces the ability of the p53 gene to work and, therefore, is more likely to allow cancers to grow. The prostate accumulates high levels of zinc, and these levels reduce greatly with cancer development (Yan, Song, Wong, Hardin, & Ho, 2008).

This is another good reason to have lots of zinc in your diet, either from food or supplementation.

In one animal experiment, progesterone was shown to reduce prostate size and weight. The researchers concluded that this study provides a basis for treating men with symptomatic BPH with progesterone (Chen, Zhou, Chen, & Kang, 1988).

As you can see, there are some good reasons to use progesterone in men with prostate disease. Progesterone supplementation for men should be about half that needed for women, approximately 1-2% progesterone cream.

ADRENALS, CORTISOL AND STRESS

"If the problem can be solved, why worry? If the problem cannot be solved, worrying will do you no good."

Shantideva, Buddhist monk (c685 CE-c763 CE)

Stress has been mentioned numerous times as a cause of, or related to, many hormone issues. Here I will discuss stress and subsequent elevated cortisol levels.

Ask any conventional doctor about adrenal disease and probably the only diseases they do know of are Cushing's disease, where the adrenal glands are working too much or Addison's disease, where the adrenal glands are not working at all. I will not look at these conditions, however, as I plan to focus on an adrenal condition that is generally not recognised by mainstream medicine.

Biology is not black and white; it is grey with only the extremes being black and white. An adrenal condition that highlights this, which is in the grey zone, and which is not Cushing's or Addison's, is "adrenal exhaustion" wherein this condition the adrenal function is suboptimal; the function can no longer meet the body's requirements.

This is a diagnosis not recognized by mainstream medicine, but this does not mean it doesn't exist.

> Adrenal exhaustion is *not* recognised by mainstream medicine.

Introduction and summary

The term "adrenal fatigue" or "adrenal exhaustion" has been debated for quite some time; (note that I have been putting "adrenal exhaustion" in inverted commas for a reason, as you shall see). This is a diagnosis being made by integrative doctors and other non-mainstream practitioners.

This diagnosis describes a collection of symptoms such as tiredness, poor immunity, sleeping difficulties, tired when waking up, unrefreshed sleep, sugar and salt craving, non-specific digestive problems, needing a coffee hit to get started, and many more. All the above are non-specific symptoms, although many symptoms are reminiscent of a low cortisol scenario. Many seem to be either produced by stress or related to stress in some way. Who does not have stress in this modern world of ours.

The original idea was that, under excessive stress, the adrenal glands become "fatigued" from overwork and couldn't produce the cortisol that was needed to keep the body functioning normally. The adrenal glands produce adrenaline and cortisol in the "fight and flight" reaction when confronted with a stressful situation.

This goes back to our paleolithic days: the scenario typically related is that our paleolithic ancestor is walking through the forest and meets up with a sabre-toothed tiger. The acute stress mechanism kicks in, initially releasing adrenaline, then the cortisol kicks in, so that our ancestor can run faster and fight harder. This is a short-term response and once he gets away, things settle down. Until the next encounter!

This same mechanism is at work now, except we do not have sabre-toothed tigers; we have bosses, tax departments, BAS, GST, poor diet, parking meters, traffic lights, traffic congestion, pollution, EMF and are "over worked and underpaid"; all of which are stressful. The same acute stress reaction kicks, but we cannot run or fight. We simply must put up with it, which probably makes it worse, as that inability to do anything about it is a cause of frustration! We could run and fight, but I do not think it would be a good idea to punch the boss. Also, today, these stressful events are more continuous; our bodies were not designed for this constant stress. Since humans have not developed a chronic stress mechanism, the body uses the acute stress mechanism repeatedly.

The studies by the Hungarian Canadian researcher Hans Selye (1907-1982) looked at the body's response to stressors, which he named the general adaptation syndrome (GAS).

He divided the GAS into 3 stages:

1) Stage 1–alarm reaction, (flight or fight),

2) Stage 2–resistance, and

3) Stage 3–exhaustion.

Some posit a stage 4–death.

The theory was extended to account for chronic stress. As with any stress, the adrenal glands work overtime to compensate for increased stress levels, and initially they cope, but eventually stress levels reaches Stage 3, exhaustion. It was this extension of the GAS theory that led to the concept of "adrenal exhaustion" also known as "adrenal fatigue". Chronic stress, it was decided, "wears out the adrenals".

This syndrome (I call it a syndrome, which means a collection of symptoms), does exist. But, as I will explain, the problem with "adrenal exhaustion" is with the underlying causative mechanism. So, in some ways, the problem is all in the name.

What is in a name?

"A rose by any other name would smell as sweet."

Romeo and Juliet, Act 2, Scene 2,
William Shakespeare (c1564 – 1616)

The various World Endocrinological Societies have never accepted the concept of "adrenal exhaustion". These societies put out statements that "adrenal fatigue" or "adrenal exhaustion" is all a load of rubbish;

they claim it to be a figment of the alternative medicine mind! They say that the adrenal glands do *not* "wear out". They do not explain any of these symptoms, although they do say that other diseases must be ruled out.

All good doctors will do this, anyway!

The complementary and integrative doctors maintain that since the diagnosis is not being recognised, the diagnosis is not being made and many people with these symptoms do not get any relief with the mainstream approach. So, those with these symptoms go to alternative practitioners, get diagnosed with "adrenal fatigue", and are treated and greatly improve.

Another condition called "burnout syndrome" is quite prominent in the psychological literature. The psychologists do not explain it or assign it any physiology or biochemistry, they just diagnose on symptoms and questionnaires.

Pranjić, Nuhbegović, Brekalo-Lazarević, and Kurtić (2012) wrote *"when workers constant expose to repeat mobbing behavior or have perception of extended distress reaction after act of violence at workplace they are suffering of Syndrome burnout and clinical picture of adrenal fatigue."*

This syndrome is largely related to stress and work. Symptomatically, there is a great overlap between the symptoms of "adrenal fatigue" and "burnout syndrome". Mainstream medicine is more accepting of "burnout syndrome" as a real thing!

Can both sides be right? To an extent–yes! Mainly because the issue is all in the name.

Above slide taken from a presentation the author gave to the Australian Medical Acupuncture College seminar in 2018.

A comprehensive study (Cadegiani & Kater, 2016) concluded that "adrenal fatigue" does not exist because all studies looked at showed that the adrenal glands do not tire out and produce less cortisol. They did detect variations in cortisol levels, low in some, high in others, although in the large majority there was not much change.

The adrenal glands are quite a robust organ, producing cortisol even after long stressful periods. So how can both sides of the argument be somewhat correct?

There is no doubt that stress affects our health.

Before we go any further, let's get back to basics and examine how the stress system works. The hypothalamus-pituitary-adrenal (HPA) axis is integral to the stress response. The HPA axis releases hormones in a circadian rhythm to regulate daily energy needs.

Corticotropin-releasing hormone (CRH) is released from the suprachiasmatic nucleus in the hypothalamus. This acts on the pituitary gland causing it to release adrenocorticotropic hormone (ACTH), which then acts on the adrenal glands causing them to release cortisol in a diurnal fashion. In normal individuals, the cortisol release is the highest in the mornings, then gradually declines by night-time, thus giving us the energy to wake up, get up and to carry out our daytime activities. Cortisol then declines by nighttime so we can fall asleep; this cycle continues day after day after day.

The amygdala is part of the brain that detects stress, physical danger, real or imagined, and then sends a signal to the hypothalamus. From here, the sympathetic nervous system sends messages via the autonomic nervous system to release adrenaline from the adrenal glands. This is the immediate stress response. Then the HPA axis kicks in via the mechanism described previously: CRH → ACTH → cortisol release, which is the more sustained response. Now, via a negative feedback mechanism, cortisol feeds back to reduce the CRH and the ACTH production. This feedback mechanism is typical of other systems in the body, such as the thyroid and TSH. This all happens in the normal situation, but we do *not* live in a "normal" situation.

What happens when there is more stress? With high stress and the constant release of cortisol, it is not that the adrenal glands "fatigue" or "tire out", but it is the HPA axis that develops the problem.

The HPA axis does not like the constant stimulation, so it "switches off". Chronically elevated cortisol levels can cause damage, so the body tries to reduce the levels. The body tries to protect itself in several ways.

One way is by developing a cortisol receptor resistance.

This also happens elsewhere.

For example, we see it in type 2 diabetes (T2D).

In T2D, it is not the pancreas that wears out. No! It is not the pancreas that fatigues, but the body develops insulin resistance. In T2D, the insulin levels can be high, not low. Can this be similar?

It is not the adrenal glands that fatigue, but it is the HPA axis and the cortisol receptors that are the site of the dysfunction.

In summary, most with "adrenal fatigue" do *not* necessarily have low "total" cortisol levels. Note that at least 80% of the cortisol is bound to corticosteroid binding globulin (CBG) and another 10% is bound to albumin. Only a small portion is unbound and "free" and it is only the "free" cortisol that is biologically active.

One popular way of measuring cortisol is with a saliva test. This only measures the "free" cortisol, not the "total" cortisol. In the past, when low cortisol levels were found on a salivary measurement, this was wrongly interpreted as the adrenals not working adequately, that they were "exhausted".

This is the wrong interpretation.

Salivary "free" cortisol may be low, but the total cortisol may be normal.

A low salivary "free" cortisol is not due to reduced production by the adrenal glands, or because they are fatigued. It is due to a down-regulation of the HPA axis. Basically, it can be viewed as a protective mechanism.

One mechanism, as mentioned above, is the development of cortisol receptor resistance (Cohen et al., 2012; Merkulov, Merkulova, & Bondar, 2017). If there is cortisol receptor resistance, cortisol cannot stimulate the receptor to achieve its action. Unfortunately, this also interferes with the cortisol feedback mechanism.

There can also be an increased level of cortisol binding globulin (CBG) which reduces the "free" cortisol by binding more (Chan, Carrell, Zhou, & Read, 2013; Mattos et al., 2013; Verhoog et al., 2014).

The level of cortisol can also be reduced by converting cortisol to cortisone. Cortisone has a much less active steroid activity. This is achieved by activation of *11 β-hydroxysteroid dehydrogenase type 2* (11β-HSD2) enzyme.

11β-HSD2 can be upregulated by interleukins such as IL-2, IL-4 and IL-13, which are increased by inflammation and in stress.

The enzyme can also be upregulated, thus increasing the conversion of active cortisol to less active cortisone by DHEA (Balazs, Schweizer, Frey, Rohner-Jeanrenaud, & Odermatt, 2008).

DHEA levels rise in acute and chronic stress, according to Morgan et al. (2004).

All this is a protective mechanism as the body tries to adapt to chronically high cortisol levels, and it may overshoot and produce a low "free" cortisol level. With the cortisol resistance, the body acts as if the cortisol is low, hence producing the typical symptoms of "low cortisol". So, it is not an "adrenal exhaustion" but an HPA axis dysregulation. While the symptoms are the same and it looks as if the adrenals are fatigued, it is the regulatory controls that are the issue, not the "fatigue" of the end organ. So, what can we call it? HPA Axis dysregulation is a mouthful–not sexy enough! HPAAD?

What causes HPA axis dysregulation?

1) Stress–real or perceived. Negative stress–distress, even good stress–eustress. Modern living, poor diet, pollution, and so on.

2) Inflammation

3) Blood sugar variations from normal–high or low

How to treat?

In some ways, the treatment is the same as for treatment of "adrenal fatigue"–how convenient!

Treatment involves the following:

1) Deal with the stress using relaxation, meditation, tai chi or chi gung, or any gentle exercise such as walking. Make changes to work, lifestyle, and diet. This is obvious but is easier said than done!

2) Deal with causes of inflammation. Treat any underlying condition, treat the gut, dysbiosis, SIBO, autoimmunity, MetS and any other problems.

3) Regulate the blood sugar level (BSL), with diet - low carb, Paleo, and incorporate fasting into your dietary routine. Regular exercise is important.

4) Get the day/night cycle back to normal. Get enough sleep, go to bed early, get up at a reasonable time, get plenty of light into the eyes during the day. Reduce the exposure to artificial lights at night. Avoid prolonged computer, iPad, iPhone exposure. Note that these devices have an overall blue colour to the screen. Blue light interferes with the production and release of the sleep hormone, melatonin. Either avoid screens completely, read a book instead, or use a programme such as "f.lux", a free downloadable programme that changes

405

the colour of the screen as the evening progresses. Some newer computer models have a similar feature already installed.

5) Supplements: use adaptogens such as ashwagandha (*Withania somnifera*). This adaptogen not only works at the adrenal level but also works at the hypothalamus level (Sengupta et al., 2018; Singh, Bhalla, de Jager, & Gilca, 2011).

Phosphatidylserine (PS) has been shown to work at the cortisol receptor level by re-sensitizing the receptor (Monteleone, Maj, Beinat, Natale, & Kemali, 1992; Hellhammer et al., 2004).

6) Acupuncture has been shown to be helpful (Wang, Zhang, & Qie, 2014; Wang, Zhang, Yang, Wang, & Li, 2015; Wei et al., 2017). Wild et al. (2020) showed benefit in a randomised controlled pilot trial.

So, after all this, we can say that the adrenals do not "wear out". We know that stress *does* have an impact on our health; producing non-specific symptoms that up until now were called "adrenal fatigue" and the symptoms are much the same as "burnout syndrome" (which is largely recognised).

As has been shown, this condition should be called "HPA axis dysregulation" - HPAAD!

The bone of contention is in the name. It is the underlying causative mechanism that should decide the name therefore, we should call it HPAAD and not "adrenal fatigue."

Tired all the time syndrome (TATTS)

Tiredness is perhaps one of the most common complaints seen in today's general medical practice. How many times do I hear the words, *"Doctor, I am so tired."*

After hearing this many times a day, I too feel tired!

There are, of course, many causes that need to be excluded, such as anaemia, iron deficiency, B12 deficiency, hypothyroidism, cancer or any other chronic disease, although when all of these are excluded, there is still a very large number of people who have TATTS; Tired All The Time Syndrome.

The reason I mention this here is that a common symptom of HPAAD is tiredness therefore conversely, HPAAD/ "adrenal exhaustion" is possibly one of the largest causes of this epidemic of tiredness: and what's more, is not recognised by the mainstream doctors.

Melding into this are other poorly defined, poorly understood syndromes, such as chronic fatigue syndrome (CFS) and fibromyalgia (FM). "Long covid" could also be added to this list. HPAAD may be a cause of CFS and FM or it may be because of CFS and FM.

The chicken or the egg scenario!

This makes sense because of the excessive amount of stress that we are exposed to in this modern western society. Some have estimated that 75-90% of all visits to a GP are related to stress in some way, and how do the mainstream GPs treat it? With various pharmaceutical products such as benzodiazepines, anti-depressants or other drugs; unfortunately, all that many GPs know is what they learned at medical school and that is to give drugs.

> *"If all you have is a hammer, everything looks like a nail."*
>
> Bernard Baruch (1870-1965)

Stress is possibly the underlying factor in many other diseases, including diabetes, cancer, heart disease, and obesity; do those conditions sound familiar? Yes, that's correct. see you remember what you have read earlier. They are a part of the metabolic syndrome (MetS). However, in the background is stress, which I have mentioned many times, in the context of diet, nutrition and lifestyle, but not in detail.

Stress is a major part of the development of MetS.

We live in a very stressful environment; and when I use the word 'stress', I am using it in the broadest sense possible. Stress is anything that puts an extra burden on the body. Stress can range from environmental factors, such as chemical pollution, EMF, power lines. to physical factors, such as heat or cold, to poor diet, to emotional factors, such as poor relationships, financial issues, tax, BAS, GST, lack of sleep, frustration with the modern world, government bureaucracy, government over-reach, government surveillance, digital ID, WHO Pandemic Treaty, central bank digital currency, the loss of cash, and so on.

Our mind is indeed a fantastic organ, it can do so much - but there is a downside. It is so fantastic, so powerful, that stress can occur even by anticipation; worrying about things that may never happen. Worrying about for example, losing your job, can be just as bad as actually losing your job.

There is even "good stress," otherwise known as

eustress. Good stress may sound like an oxymoron but let me paint you a word picture. Imagine you are going on a holiday to Bali, or Thailand, or some other exotic destination. There is the stress of leaving Australia, organizing the tickets, making sure your passport is still valid, then making a last-minute dash to the passport office because it has expired, then the packing, organizing friends and relatives to look after the house while you are away, to feed the dog, to water the garden; is this stressful? Well, yes, it is, but it is good stress because you are going on a holiday.

> *"Adopting the right attitude can convert a negative stress into a positive one."*
>
> Hans Selye (1907–1982)

As you can see, there is a very wide range of things that can be classified under "stress".

The act of being born is stressful. And as soon as we are born, we are subjected to a polluted world full of chemicals, insecticides, plastics, petrol and diesel fumes, and many other toxins, all of which put a burden on our bodies.

Another source of stress is the diet. Many babies are fed an artificial diet based on "foreign to human" proteins: cow's milk. We grow up, we must go to school, we have to study, in many ways, in a very artificial situation. There are many rules and laws we must follow, many which do not make sense; I could go on and on. Hopefully, by now, that you get the idea. These situations are foreign to our species. During our evolution, until recent history, things were much simpler. The stress our ancestors experienced was mostly an *acute* stress that lasted a relatively short time, not the prolonged stress we are now subject to.

There is a scenario that is often recounted to reflect the above. Our paleolithic ancestor is walking through the forest and meets up with a sabre-toothed tiger. This is acute stress. The organism developed a mechanism to deal with the situation: the "fight or flight" response. Adrenaline and cortisol are released allowing our paleolithic ancestor to run faster or fight harder. If he ran faster or fought harder and survived, the stress settled and didn't worry about it until the next time. If he wasn't successful, then a dead person does not evolve any chronic stress mechanisms!

So, we have mechanisms to cope with short-term stress, but our species did not develop a mechanism to deal with long- term stress. The body tries to use the short-term mechanism to deal with a chronic situation, which works to a degree, but eventually the system collapses.

In 1946, Hans Selye described this stress response and introduced the general adaptive syndrome (GAS).

We humans can adapt to many situations and can cope for varying periods of time. Some may only last for days, others can cope for years, but eventually Stage 3 exhaustion, is reached. This phase may last for shorter or longer periods until finally Stage 4 is reached: death.

> *"It's not the stress that kills us, it's our reaction to it."*
>
> Hans Selye (1907–1982)

Cortisol secretion

To keep this discussion simple, I will focus mainly on the hormone cortisol. A more complicated discussion on stress can be found in the book, 'Why Zebras Don't Get Ulcers' (Sapolsky, 1994).

One function of the adrenal glands is to release cortisol; however, it is not just *how much* cortisol is released, but also *when* it is released.

Cortisol has a normal diurnal cycle, where cortisol levels are highest in the morning, then reduces during the day and is the lowest at midnight. Cortisol is an energy hormone, so it makes sense that the peak is in the morning. This energy is needed for us to wake up and to get going in the morning. The morning cortisol peak kick-starts the day.

People complaining of HPAAD/ "adrenal exhaustion" need to be diagnosed properly, and this can only be done by

1) knowing about the condition, and
2) measuring their cortisol levels, both "free" and "total."

Blood cortisol levels do not give a full picture for this situation, for similar reasons given for blood levels not being accurate when measuring sex hormones.

A frequently used test is the 24-hour urinary cortisol. On one hand, this is a good test because it shows the total amount of cortisol produced in a day, but on the other hand, is also inadequate because it does not give us information about the timing. For example, a low morning cortisol with a high afternoon cortisol could still produce a normal 24-hour cortisol urinary output. This is not helpful.

Another way to measure adrenal function is to do salivary cortisol levels at 0600-0700, 1200, 1800 and 2200. This method measures "free" cortisol only. "Free" cortisol can be altered by various ways as previously discussed. Remember, with sex hormones, especially testosterone, the level of "free" biologically active testosterone is dependent on SHBG. CBG is not measured routinely and is difficult to arrange and generally not done.

Why saliva? As with sex hormones, steroid hormones work intra-cellularly. We want to know tissue levels of the hormone, not what may be floating around in the blood. Saliva is ideal for this. Also, as with sex hormones, there is a binding protein, so to bypass the difficulties with the binding proteins, saliva levels are more useful.

Laudat et al. (1988) wrote that *"We conclude that salivary cortisol measurements are an excellent index of plasma free cortisol concentrations. They circumvent the physiological, pathological, and pharmacological changes due to corticosteroid-binding globulin alterations and offer a practical approach to assess pituitary-adrenal function."*

In this context, we are measuring the cortisol to look at it from a functional point of view, to see how well it is working.

In the initial phases, the levels of "free" cortisol may be high, before HPAAD sets in, when there may be too little. In other situations, the adrenal glands may release the correct amount, but at the wrong time.

We can therefore predict that if the morning peak is absent or reduced, people will wake up tired. Even after a good night's sleep, a person with HPAAD will wake up tired. How often do you hear people complaining that they wake up tired despite sleeping all night? Now you know why?

Another scenario is when people wake up tired, but by the evening, they may be wide awake, can't relax and are anxious. They cannot sleep. They eventually fall asleep at three or four in the morning, then wake up tired. How often do you hear this?

Tired in the morning and insomnia at night. "Tired" and "wired". This is also a very common scenario. Cortisol is too low in the mornings and too high at night. We should treat the adrenal glands/HPA axis, not just trying to cover up the symptom with the use of strong sleeping tablets.

A common feature is that all these people are under some form of chronic stress. As part of history taking, ask about their past. All sorts of thing will come out: bad childhood, parents' divorce, sexual molestation,

415

bullying at school, bad marriage, chronic illness, work issues, financial issues, ("over-worked and under-paid"); the list could go on.

Note that stress in the past can still produce issues in the present. With some, once the past stress is over, things settle down. With others, past stress, especially childhood stress conditions, tends to stay for a very long time.

There may be a precipitating incident, where the present medical problems started after an acute episode of stress, an acute illness, an operation, a car accident, childbirth, the death of a loved one, and so on.

With some, there is a temporary "adrenal dysfunction" which normalises once the stress has settled. With others, the adrenal/HPA axis dysfunction gets stuck in the abnormal pattern. Why? We do not know for sure.

All these scenarios are because of HPA axis dysfunction. Initially there may be excess "free" cortisol, then the next phase is reduced "free" cortisol, without an actual reduction in total cortisol release, and somewhere in between, there may be inappropriate release.

Treatment involves getting the "free" cortisol levels to a more normal pattern.

Stress chips away at HPA axis function. With some, the symptoms come on quickly, with others it may take time, but eventually everyone has a point where the HPA axis/adrenal system will become dysfunctional.

Symptoms of HPAAD/ "adrenal exhaustion"

We have mentioned that the main symptom of HPAAD is tiredness. We can be a bit more specific and say inappropriate tiredness. Being tired at the end of a hard day's work can be normal and appropriate. Having your energy cycle out of sync, being tired in the morning and wide awake at night, is not normal.

Low blood pressure is another prominent symptom and can be used as a diagnostic test. Dizziness on standing up, or becoming dizzy on prolonged standing, is related to this. Generally, on standing up, BP goes up, but with HPAAD, BP goes down (postural hypotension). We can use this clinically. Measure a person's BP sitting and standing and see if there is any change.

Some people lose weight, others gain weight, and still others seem unable to lose weight despite trying to. This is related to the thyroid-adrenal connection. If you remember our discussion of Addison's disease, you will remember that weight loss is a major symptom. In

417

Cushing's disease, the problem is weight gain.

Salt craving is related to the "cortisol steal" that was mentioned earlier. If the biochemical highway is all the way to cortisol, there is little to go to the side pathway to aldosterone, which is the hormone that reabsorbs salt and water from the kidneys. Lack of this hormone causes increased urination and loss of salt, so people pee a lot (have you noticed that people rush off to the toilet when stressed?), including getting up at night frequently to pee (nocturia) and therefore, they become salt deficient and crave salt. In men, another reason for nocturia is prostate problems.

The cortisol steal also has the same effect on DHEA; it reduces levels, which leads to sex hormone problems

Low blood sugars and sugar craving are also symptoms and are related to the blood sugar regulation of cortisol.

Overall, people respond poorly to stress. They simply can't cope, not only with emotional issues but physical issues as well. When under stress, even the little things that never used to bother a person in the past can seem insurmountable. Increased frustration, constant anger, yelling, road rage, and decreased tolerance are related to an inability to manage stress. Drug use, smoking and alcohol–self-medicating, are all ways of trying to reduce the stress. However, as we know, this probably causes more harm than help. A glass of wine with dinner after a hard day at the office, however, can be beneficial. A whole bottle is not!

People also complain of catching cold easily (poor immune system) and that it takes weeks to recover. The whole family gets a runny nose, the stressed one gets double pneumonia!

In the fight-or-flight response, blood is shunted from the pelvic area to the muscles to enable a person to run faster and fight harder. When you are fighting or running away from a predator or enemy, sex is not a priority. This leads to poor libido, sexual difficulties, PMT and menstrual problems.

During the fight or flight, blood is shunted away from the gut to the muscles for running faster or fighting harder. Digestion is also not a priority when fighting or running away. This leads to digestive issues and gut problems.

Diarrhoea can be a sign of stress. If you are a zebra being chased by a lion, a quick evacuation of the bowels will make you lighter and you can run faster. The lion may also get a face full of faeces, which hopefully may slow it down! Conversely, the bowel peristalsis can become so un-coordinated that there is no net forward movement, therefore constipation may develop.

There may be a late afternoon pick up, the "second wind", meaning that the afternoon is probably the best they feel all day.

Fuzzy thinking, or poor memory, can develop.

Life becomes a drag, so there is no enjoyment in life and even a mild depression may develop.

Symptoms may be aggravated by missing a meal.

Women may have extra severe PMT, or they may have all sorts of hormonal problems, ranging from amenorrhoea to period irregularity to infertility.

Insomnia may also be a problem, especially if the cortisol levels are high at night. There is a see-saw relationship between cortisol and melatonin. If cortisol is high, melatonin is low. A high nocturnal cortisol interferes with a good night's sleep.

There are some who try melatonin for sleep but say that it doesn't help. Because of the cortisol/melatonin see-saw, when there is a high cortisol level, there needs to be an extra-large dose of melatonin to reduce the cortisol levels and then this will bring on sleep. A pharmaceutical company makes a 2 mg tablet, compounding pharmacists can make higher dose capsules. While many are reluctant to take high doses, with appropriate advice, they will be more confident in doing so, at least initially. Melatonin dosage may need to be as high as 10 mg or more, to influence the high cortisol levels. Melatonin is effective at reducing cortisol levels.

If you look at the above list, the symptoms are quite broad but when taken into context of a tired person who has had a lot of stress in their life, then the diagnosis is worth considering.

Physical examination may be non-contributory, but there are two clinical tests that may give a clue. One has already been mentioned. A drop in BP when the person stands up (postural hypotension). Or just a low BP. They often remark, *"My local doctor always says I have a low BP."*

Another useful sign is an unstable pupillary reflex. Generally, if a light is shined into the eyes, the pupils will contract and remain contracted while the light is shining. In HPAAD, the pupil contracts at first, then dilates, then can continue to contract and dilate. The explanation is that, since there is muscle weakness and tiredness, even the muscles in the iris cannot sustain prolonged constriction, they tire out and relax, therefore dilating the pupil. Many complain that sun-glare bothers them, and they need to wear sunglasses continually. This makes sense, as the pupil cannot remain constricted in the sunlight.

If I see a patient who has their sunglasses on their head, I refer to this as "Baratosy's sign": named after myself! This is especially significant in Tasmania, where I practice. When patients who tell me that they wear their sunnies even in mid-winter, it is especially suggestive of the need for further assessment.

How to treat?

Treatment is simple, as realistically there are only two things to do; raise the "free" cortisol if too low or reduce it if it is too high.

However, it may not always be as simple as that.

I use the analogy of the balcony. Over the last few months there have been stories in the papers, where at a party or function, a balcony has collapsed, and many people have been injured.

What has this to do with HPAAD?

Simple.

To prevent a balcony from collapsing, two things can be done:

1) reduce the number of people on the balcony and/or
2) support the balcony.

You can see the analogy (I hope).

To treat HPAAD, you first must reduce the stress on the person and secondly support the adrenal glands/HPA axis.

Stress reduction is easier said than done. There are stresses you can reduce with proper advice or by changing your situation. There are stresses you cannot change easily. Changing your job is not easy, although there are some who have changed to a lower-paying job and have found it worthwhile, as they are happy and less stressed.

Learning to meditate or practice yoga or tai chi can be a help. Put aside some "you" time. Take temporary breaks away from the situation: go to the pictures, have a massage, have a coffee and a chat with a friend. Go for a walk and hug a tree.

Food allergies/intolerances can be a hidden form of stress, so dietary change to a low stress diet can help. Nutritional advice can assist when making this change.

423

If it is a bad marriage, either get counselling or a divorce lawyer! If it is financial stress, get advice from an accountant, talk to your creditors, some plan can always be negotiated.

Worrying about a situation, e.g. losing your job, can cause precisely the same amount of stress as if you actually lost your job. Of course, saying "don't worry" is easier than doing it!

"Don't worry... be happy."

Bobby McFerrin (1988)

Every single person with stress has their own unique situation, and it needs to be dealt with as an individual.

Essentially you need to look at your stress and know what you can change and what you cannot. If you can change it; then do so. If you cannot change it; then do the things mentioned to support yourself.

Support the adrenals and the HPA axis

There are different ways to support your adrenals and HPA axis. Some have already been mentioned and these revolve around reducing and minimising your stress. Getting the excess people off your balcony!

The other way to help yourself is to support your balcony by helping and supporting your adrenal glands and HPA axis. This can be done by taking various herbs, nutrients, and supplements. Note, of course, that this does not remove your stress; it just helps you to cope better!

Herbs

1) Liquorice

Liquorice comes from the root of the plant *Glycyrrhiza glabra*. The liquorice plant is related to beans and peas and is native to southern Europe and parts of Asia. Liquorice contains a compound called glycyrrhizin that has an inhibiting effect on the enzyme *11β-hydroxysteroid dehydrogenase (type 2)*. This enzyme normally inactivates cortisol in the kidney by converting cortisol to cortisone, a less active steroid. Liquorice inhibits this enzyme, therefore raising the level of cortisol in the body by inhibiting its conversion.

425

Cortisol acts at the same receptor as the hormone aldosterone in the kidney and the effects mimic aldosterone excess, although aldosterone remains low. Liquorice also has the effect of raising blood pressure (BP) which can be considered a dangerous side effect. However, since people with HPAAD generally have low BP, this may initially be advantageous. Continued use, though, may produce an elevated blood pressure, which may have a negative effect and therefore anyone on long-term liquorice should have their BP regularly monitored. A common dosage is 2-3 grams of liquorice root twice a day. Use it for a maximum of eight weeks before tapering off the dosage, otherwise you may raise the cortisol levels too high and cause high blood pressure as well as interfering with fluid balance,

2) Ginseng (*Panax spp.*)

There are eleven distinct species belonging to the Panax family, which grows mainly in eastern Asia (mostly northern China, Korea, and eastern Siberia), typically in cooler climates; The standard Asian ginseng is *Panax ginseng. Panax vietnamensis*, discovered in Vietnam, is the most southernmost ginseng found, while American ginseng (*Panax quinquefolius*) as the name implies, grows in the USA. "Siberian ginseng" (*Eleutherococcus senticosus*) is not a true ginseng but was called "Siberian ginseng" mainly for marketing purposes. Withania (see below) is often referred to as Indian ginseng. This also is not a true ginseng.

Ginseng, in herbal terms, is classed as an adaptogen. The term adaptogen is used by herbalists to refer to a herb that increases the body's resistance to stress, trauma, anxiety and fatigue. Adaptogens generally normalise the function of the HPA axis.

3) *Withania*

Withania somnifera, also known as ashwagandha, Indian ginseng or winter cherry, is a plant in the Solanaceae or nightshade family, and is also considered an adaptogen. An adaptogen is an herb that works to normalize physiological function, working on the HPA axis and the neuroendocrine system. Although it is called Indian ginseng, it is not a true ginseng, though has similar properties.

Many of the herbal companies (I will not name any specific companies or products) produce an adrenal support formula which contains some or all these herbs, as well as some of the nutrients mentioned below.

Phosphatidylserine

Phosphatidylserine (PS) is a phospholipid that is used in cell membranes and has been shown to reduce excess cortisol levels by repairing the cortisol receptors in the hypothalamus or by blunting the release of cortisol. To explain simply, PS repairs the cortisol thermostat. There seems to be some evidence that PS can also be useful in low cortisol states (Monteleone, Beinat, Tanzillo, Maj, & Kemali, 1990; Monteleone, Maj, Beinat, Natale, & Kemali,1992).

PS is also useful in short-term memory loss, age related dementia and Alzheimer's disease.

Dosage 100mg up to three times a day.

A related phospholipid, phosphatidylcholine (PC), generally known as lecithin, does not have these same properties.

Of course, if levels of cortisol are too high, they need to be reduced with the herbs, nutrients and stress-reduction methods already mentioned.

If cortisol levels are too low, then they can be stimulated with the nutrients and herbs mentioned above, as well as with stress reduction. The herbs and nutrients may take some months to start to work.

Nutrients

Before I mention specific nutrients, we should look at diet. A good diet, or should I say–eating pattern, is essential if one is to recover from HPAAD. The diet should be nutritious and produce a low stress for the body. Here, we go back to the "low stress diet". (It is called low stress for a reason!) This eating pattern is low in refined carbohydrates, sugar, coffee, alcohol, preservatives, colours, and flavourings. We have already looked at this diet.

There are some nutrients that are specifically required for adrenal support. These are vitamin C, B complex–especially B5, zinc and magnesium.

1) Vitamin C

I have written a lot about vitamin C in previous books. Here, I will focus specifically on the role of vitamin C in adrenal function.

Vitamin C is perhaps the most important factor needed in adrenal metabolism. Vitamin C is essential in the production of cortisol, so much so that before the introduction of cortisol assays, vitamin C measurement was used as the best indicator of cortisol production in animal research.

Just a piece of trivia: on a weight for weight basis, the adrenal glands contain the highest concentration of vitamin C in the body.

The more stress, the more cortisol is manufactured, the more vitamin C is used up. Doses must be supplemented in sizable quantities; and here I am talking about grams, not milligrams. In nature bioflavonoids always accompany vitamin C, so ideally it is always better to eat fresh fruit than to take a supplement. However, vitamin C deteriorates as soon as the fruit is picked from the tree. Therefore, fruit stored for months in cool rooms, fruit picked green and allowed to ripen in the box on the back of a truck, or worse still, green fruit artificially ripened by exposing it to chemical gasses all result in very poor levels of vitamin C. The only practical way to get a decent dose of vitamin C is to supplement. You can still eat fruit for the bioflavonoid content!

What is the best form of vitamin C supplement?

I recommend sodium ascorbate powder. This is a pure form without colours, flavours, or preservatives. One level teaspoon of sodium ascorbate powder is approximately 4.5 grams of vitamin C.

Vitamin C tablets contain colours, flavours, sweeteners (saccharin, aspartame, etc), and preservatives, binders and fillers. To get a decent dose, many tablets are needed. To avoid the ingestion of these unwanted chemicals, it is best to avoid the tablets.

How much do you need to take?

Perhaps the most optimal way to decide what is the maximum dose for everyone is to use the concept of the "bowel tolerance". Slowly increase the dose until your bowel actions become runny, then cut back to a level where there are no bowel effects.

Vitamin C also has a positive effect on the immune system, so this is a second reason to take vitamin C.

2) B complex

How often has it been said that stress "uses up" vitamin B complex? There is some truth to this. Certainly, from a clinical perspective stressed people who take a B complex do feel better.

Why?

Here again we must look at the biochemistry.

B complex and especially B_5 (pantothenic acid) is probably the most important. B_5 is converted to acetyl CoA, which is needed for energy production. This is needed in all cells, but more is needed in the adrenal glands because of the energy required to make all the cortisol.

Do not take B₅ only … you must take a B complex as well. The B group vitamins are like bees, they work together in a swarm!

3) Magnesium

This mineral is essential for energy production, not just in the adrenal glands, but in all cells. Magnesium (Mg) is a co-factor needed for over 300 enzyme reactions. The unfortunate thing is that a large proportion of the western word is deficient, largely relating to the high incidence of MetS as discussed earlier

Mg is one of those essential minerals that is needed to drive not just the adrenal cortisol cascade but is essential for energy production as well.

The recommended maximum oral dose is 6 mg per kilogram body weight per day. However, note that Mg absorption through the gut is dependent on vitamin D. Another way to supplement Mg is to bypass the gut and supplement it transdermally. You can do this by soaking in a bath of Epsom salts (magnesium sulphate) or applying it in the form of magnesium chloride ($MgCl_2$)

which is now available as a topical cream, gel or oil.

A long hot soak in an Epsom Salts bath is stress relieving in itself!

4) Zinc

Zinc (Zn) is another important co-factor for over 200 enzyme reactions, including in the production of cortisol. Conversely, high cortisol levels can reduce Zn levels. Zn is also needed to improve immune function, which we now know is reduced in HPAAD. The role of Zn in adrenal function is very complicated. Here we have a two-way process. Cortisol can control Zn metabolism, and Zn affects cortisol production. Animal studies have shown that Zn deficient rats had heavier adrenal glands than normal rats. *"The increased adrenal lipid composition in the zinc deficient group may be secondary to enhanced steroidogenesis or a zinc deficiency-induced defect of lipid metabolism"* (Rothman, Leure-duPree, & Fosmire, 1986).

Conversely, Zn supplementation can lower cortisol secretion, by producing an acute inhibitory effect on cortisol secretion (Brandão-Neto et al., 1990).

Things get even more complicated.

Cortisol enhances Zn uptake, which stimulates the expression of metallothionein and Zn transporter-1 genes. Although note that this was done with an animal model: rainbow trout. (Bury, Chung, Sturm, Walker, & Hogstrand, 2008).

Metallothionein (MT) is a protein that can bind physiological minerals such as Zn, copper (Cu) and selenium (Se), as well as toxic HMs such as mercury (Hg), cadmium (Cd) and arsenic (As). MT is involved in regulation of the physiological metals such as Zn, as well as acting as a storage mechanism for the HMs. MT is a major protein in the storage and transport of Zn in the body. HMs can also bind to MT and therefore can displace Zn or other physiological metals. Now you can appreciate why HMs have such a profound blocking effect on normal metabolism of Zn (or other physiological metals). MT is very important in brain function where Zn signalling is integral in communication between and within nerve cells. MT also seems to have an important role in the regulation of the p53 gene.

Zn, as well as Cd, can stimulate the production of MT (Wan, Hunziker, & Kägi, 1993). Zn, Cd and Hg are in the same column on the periodic table, and therefore have some similar properties.

There also seems to be a feed-back loop. Low Zn causes an increase in cortisol, which enhances Zn absorption, which then can reduce cortisol production. This would be important in the regulation of Zn levels but could be an issue if there is an actual Zn deficiency.

There is a see-saw relationship between Zn and Cu. When Cu is high, Zn is low and *vice versa.* The reason I mention this is because of the heavy use of Cu today; copper pipes, copper used in water treatment (copper sulphate), copper used in agriculture as a fungicide, and so on.

One sign of a high Cu is anxiety. The enzyme that converts dopamine to noradrenaline, *dopamine beta-hydroxylase (DBH)*, is a Cu dependant enzyme. A relative excess of Cu can stimulate this enzyme.

Also note that a high Cu means there is a low Zn. The production of gamma amino butyric acid (GABA), the "calm you down neurotransmitter" relies on Zn and B_6.

We are also living in a sea of oestrogens and/or xenoestrogens. Oestrogens tend to cause Cu retention. There is too much copper, therefore Zn may be low. Zn supplementation should be up to 30 mg per day on average but in some may need to go higher.

The best source of Zn is meat. This is one reason

vegetarians have low Zn levels. Oysters are a good source, and this is the possible reason why oysters are regarded as an aphrodisiac; high Zn content helps sexual function.

As one of my patients complained to me: he said that ate a dozen oysters and only four of them worked!

Although I have mentioned only a few specific nutrients, many who have HPAAD have other issues and are possibly deficient in multiple nutrients. This is where a thorough history and examination taken by a nutritional doctor, especially one trained by the Australasian College of Nutritional and Environmental Medicine (ACNEM) will show what other minerals may be missing.

In the early stages of HPAAD, the levels of "free" cortisol may be high as the body tries to deal with the stress. These high levels of cortisol have adverse effects. High cortisol levels can influence thyroid function and can also interfere with the sex hormones.

First, there may be a reduction of progesterone manufacture due to the "cortisol steal" phenomenon.

Then, there is some crosstalk between cortisol and progesterone receptors due to their similarity and a high cortisol may have a blocking effect by competing with progesterone at the receptor level (Leo, Guo, Woon, Aw,

& Lin, 2004).

Karalis, Goodwin, and Majzoub (1996) looked at factors that bring on birth in animals, which may also apply to humans. The level of progesterone does not drop but there is an increase in cortisol from the foetus and the researchers concluded that the cortisol blocks the progesterone receptors, which then brings on birth.

If this is correct and cortisol blocks progesterone receptors not only during pregnancy, then this mechanism will cause menstrual problems which we see during stress. Also, stress may inhibit pregnancy through this mechanism.

Cortisol replacement therapy (CRT)

Cortisol replacement is akin to HRT, or hormone replacement therapy. We can call it cortisol replacement therapy (CRT). In some situations, e.g. Addison's disease, this is the only way to increase cortisol levels.

Since the adrenal glands do not get "exhausted," the use of cortisol replacement is not generally suggested. In the past, "adrenal exhaustion" was treated with CRT, and in retrospect, many did not gain the benefit that had been hoped for. However, there were some who responded very well.

One clue: ask if they have ever been prescribed steroids for any other condition, e.g. for asthma, and if they report that there was a positive response to their tiredness when using the steroids, then a trial of CRT can be commenced.

Note: This is not Plan A. Use the herbs and nutrients first.

A comparison can be made with the use of insulin in the treatment of T2D, and the use of cortisol in the treatment of HPAAD. We know that in T2D the problem is not a lack of insulin, insulin may be elevated. The underlying problem is a reduction of insulin function due to insulin resistance. Similarly, in HPAAD, where there is cortisol receptor resistance, a short course of cortisol may be considered when all else has failed.

Once we have made the diagnosis and have shown with salivary cortisol levels that there is low morning "free" cortisol, and we have excluded other diseases, then we can commence treatment.

Of course, the first step is to discuss with the patient a change from their current diet to a low stress diet, then a plan is made for supplementing with the relevant herbs and nutrients. And important in the plan the patient makes, is how they will complement the diet, herbs and nutrients, with stress reducing activities in whatever ways is appropriate for them.

Once the doctor decides that CRT should be trialled, this is discussed with the patient.

When CRT is first mentioned, the average patient becomes frightened and even concerned. This makes sense as the general population is well aware of the negative side effects of steroids. To most people cortisol is the same as steroids. In fact, it is not unusual to hear people referring to any steroid as cortisol. For example, someone who has a shoulder problem will often say they are having a "cortisol shot". This is not correct as we have seen in the first half of the book. So, as there is a lack of awareness of the difference between 'cortisol' and steroids, many justifiably worry that they may end up like others they know who have been taking steroids of some kind. They have seen relatives, friends or neighbours who have put on weight, developed infections easily, whose skin has stretched, and whose faces became balloon-like. They are afraid this will happen to them.

It is important to reassure them that we are giving cortisol, which is the natural hormone made by all healthy people and we are giving only a low dose.

The next thing is that we must explain that the side effects they have seen in others are a consequence of taking the synthetic steroids, such as prednisolone or dexamethasone. These are much more powerful than natural cortisol, especially when given in high (supra-physiological) doses. They are given to sick people to suppress the inflammation in their bodies.

At rest, the adrenal glands can make about 25 mg of cortisol a day. Under stress, it can increase to over 200 mg a day.

In Australia, there is a bio-identical cortisol available on the Pharmaceutical Benefits Scheme (PBS). This means it is subsidized by the Australian Government, so is relatively cheap. This product is hydrocortisone, which is the same as cortisol. It comes as a 4 mg or a 25 mg tablet.

Cortisone replacement therapy (CRT) must start low and should not exceed 25 mg a day, without good reason.

I would generally start with 2 x 4 mg tablets (= 8 mg) in the morning and can increase by half tablets to a maximum of 4 tablets (= 16 mg) if needed and depending on how they feel. The tablets need to be taken first thing in the morning to mimic the morning cortisol peak.

Occasionally, especially if the levels are especially low, another tablet can be taken in the middle of the day, but no more. We do not want a high cortisol level in the evening, as that would interfere with sleep.

The general principle is to give the higher dose in the morning and a lower dose in the middle of the day and the smallest dose at night.

Improvements may be noted relatively quickly.

Some have questioned this practice and certainly other doctors, especially endocrinologists, who do not recognise "adrenal exhaustion" are very negative about this.

Can I prove that this does work and is safe?

Yes.

I will take one step back here. One of the most common symptoms of HPAAD is tiredness and/or exhaustion. There are many people with these symptoms, and many have been diagnosed as chronic fatigue syndrome (CFS). The more I look at these people, the more I think that HPAAD is either a cause of their problem or is, at least, a large part of their condition.

Low cortisol levels (hypocortisolism) have been found to be associated with CFS. So, if I quote studies on CFS, you will see how it may fit into the picture.

Cleare et al. (2001) studied the use of low dose cortisol in CFS. The researchers wrote, *"We conclude that the improvement in fatigue seen in some patients with chronic fatigue syndrome during hydrocortisone treatment is accompanied by a reversal of the blunted cortisol responses to human CRH."*

Note: CRH = corticotropin-releasing hormone. This hormone is released from the hypothalamus and stimulates the pituitary to release adrenocorticotropin hormone (ACTH) which in turn stimulates the adrenal glands to release cortisol.

Baschetti (2003) commented that CFS can be thought of as a form of Addison's disease. He observed that CFS and Addison's disease share thirty-nine features: too many to be just a coincidence. He also made the comment that, like Addison's disease, the treatment of CFS can be by supplementing cortisol.

Previous reports have shown mild hypocortisolism in patients with CFS, so Cleare et al. (1999) treated a group of people diagnosed with CFS with hydrocortisone (note: hydrocortisone is the same as cortisol) for one month and then placebo for one month in a random crossover method. The researchers concluded that *"In some patients with chronic fatigue syndrome, low-dose hydrocortisone reduces fatigue levels in the short term. Treatment for a longer time and follow-up studies are needed to find out whether this effect could be clinically useful."*

McKenzie et al. (1998) showed that hydrocortisone (cortisol) replacement *"was associated with some improvement in symptoms of CFS"* however, they made the comment that the *"degree of adrenal suppression precludes its practical use for CFS."*

Some of these patients deteriorated and their cortisol levels dropped even lower due to adrenal suppression.

First, one comment: CFS is a poorly understood condition and there is no specific treatment available. Any treatment that can improve the condition should be considered.

The other comment to make is that if you look at the doses used in the McKenzie et al. (1998) study, they were over 25 mg per day. This higher dose is probably the reason for the observed adrenal suppression.

The study by Cleare et al. (1999) used *lower* doses (25 mg or less) and these were shown to be safe. This dosage does *not* suppress the HPA axis and there is no concern if the cortisol needs to be stopped.

Anyone on long-term steroids has a problem with HPA axis suppression and it is important that steroids are

443

reduced slowly.

Low dose cortisol does not seem to have this problem. Low dose cortisol can be stopped relatively quickly if necessary.

The long-term use of cortisol does not need to be a concern as the plan generally involves only temporary use, to give symptomatic relief while waiting for the herbs, nutrients, and other stress reduction strategies to start to have their action.

The above studies did not use herbs, nutrients, diet or stress reducing techniques.

CRT is a short-term therapy with the aim of reducing stress to a manageable level, then ceasing it because it has done its job. The herbs, nutrients, and other strategies will continue to do the work that CRT began.

Occasionally, the cortisol cannot be stopped because the symptoms return. Should this happen, we must weigh up the benefits of a better quality of life, with giving long-term low doses of cortisol.

A good reference is *"Safe Uses of Cortisol"* Third Edition by William McK Jefferies MD, FACP, Publ. Charles C Thomas 2004.

Thyroid-adrenal connection

I have already mentioned of the thyroid-adrenal connection in the first half of the book. These glands do not work in isolation; they help each other. From a clinical perspective you categorically should treat both, the thyroid, and the adrenals.

Adrenal effects on the thyroid

Cortisol influences thyroid function at four levels: not only at the hypothalamic and pituitary levels but also at the gland itself and at the periphery.

Stress, which has shown to increase cortisol, has a powerful impact on thyroid function.

One important action is the effect on the release of TSH. Higher cortisol levels reduce the production of TSH at the pituitary level, produce a blunted response to TSH in the gland itself and influence the peripheral conversion of inactive thyroid hormone (T4) to the active form (T3).

"CRH plays an important role in inhibiting GnRH secretion during stress, while, via somatostatin, it also inhibits GH, TRH and TSH secretion, suppressing, thus, the reproductive, growth and thyroid functions." "The

end-hormones of the hypothalamic–pituitary–adrenal (HPA) axis, glucocorticoids, on the other hand, have multiple roles. They simultaneously inhibit the CRH, LC/NE and β-endorphin systems and stimulate the mesocorticolimbic dopaminergic system and the CRH peptidergic central nucleus of the amygdala. In addition, they directly inhibit pituitary gonadotropin, GH and TSH secretion, render the target tissues of sex steroids and growth factors resistant to these substances and suppress the 5' deiodinase, which converts the relatively inactive tetraiodothyronine (T_4) to triiodothyronine (T_3), contributing further to the suppression of reproductive, growth and thyroid functions. They also have direct as well as insulin-mediated effects on adipose tissue, ultimately promoting visceral adiposity, insulin resistance, dyslipidemia and hypertension (metabolic syndrome X) and direct effects on the bone, causing "low turnover" osteoporosis" (Tsigos & Chrousos, 2002).

The cortisol levels do not have to be huge. Even mild elevation of endogenous cortisol, such as caused by fasting, can reduce serum TSH levels (Samuels & McDaniel, 1997).

Why is this important?

Perhaps I should ask: *"How is thyroid function measured conventionally?"*

Mainstream medicine relies heavily on blood TSH levels to determine thyroid function. They regard it as the "gold standard". If you consider what has just been said, can we solely rely on TSH levels? If TSH is influenced by cortisol, how relevant is the measurement of TSH?

Can we interpret the TSH level without knowing cortisol levels, or at least taking them into account? Remember that any sick person is stressed, and the cortisol levels are elevated.

Many obviously clinically hypothyroid patients have been diagnosed as "normal" because their TSH is "normal". I would ask, why is the TSH "normal" and not elevated? Could it be because the high cortisol is interfering with TSH release?

Cortisol also has an effect at the periphery.

The thyroid gland releases all the circulating inactive thyroid hormone (T4), as well as releasing some active thyroid hormone (T3). For the thyroid hormone (T4) to have its action at the periphery, it needs to be activated to T3. Cortisol has been shown to reduce the conversion of T4 to T3. (Kelly, 2000; Bános, Takó, Salamon, Györgyi, & Czikkely,1979).

When there is an elevated cortisol, T4 is preferentially converted to reverse T3 (rT3), which is a wholly inactive form of thyroid hormone. Therefore, even though TSH may be normal and T4 levels may be normal, T3 may be low because of the reduction of T4 to T3 conversion.

"... rT3 is a more potent inhibitor of T4 to T3 conversion than propylthiouracil (PTU) which is a medication used to decrease thyroid function in hyperthyroidism. In fact, rT3 is 100 times more potent than PTU at reducing T4 to T3 conversion" (Chopra, 1977).

Measuring rT3 should be a part of a full thyroid investigation.

T3 levels should also be regularly measured. Unfortunately, many mainstream doctors do not measure this. There may be clinical hypothyroidism, despite normal TSH and T4.

Another hormone that is produced by the adrenal glands is DHEA.

DHEA levels have been shown to be low with "adrenal exhaustion" caused by the "cortisol steal phenomenon". DHEA can be considered a de facto measurement of adrenal function. In the first half of the book, I discuss the use of DHEA, and although the true function is not known for sure, low levels in people who are symptomatic with CFS, or HPAAD may benefit from replacement.

One reason for the importance of DHEA is because of its relationship to T3. Both T3 and DHEA are needed at the mitochondrial receptor level to work properly to produce energy (Su & Lardy, 1991).

Thyroid effect on the adrenal

Consider a person with undiagnosed, or even borderline hypothyroidism; what is this doing to the body?

Doesn't the reduced level of thyroid hormone put extra stress on the body?

Since the thyroid hormone is the main hormone that regulates metabolic rate, wouldn't a low thyroid hormone level also slow down the adrenal glands?

Yes, but since the job of the adrenal glands is to fight stress and try to increase energy, won't they have to work harder to make up for the low thyroid state?

Wouldn't this also "exhaust" the adrenal glands even faster?

From a clinical perspective, when first treating a case of hypothyroidism, it makes sense to start by also supporting the adrenal glands. Most thyroid support products also contain an adrenal herb, such as ashwagandha.

Anxiety, phobias, post-traumatic stress disorder (PTSD) and panic attacks

Anxiety disorders are becoming very common in today's modern western society.

Why?

Could it be due to the stress and the developing HPAAD?

Quite possibly.

This notion makes sense. After all, stress and adrenal function are inter-related. What happens when the stress comes, and the body cannot respond adequately or appropriately?

Studies have shown that cortisol levels are important in the genesis of anxiety disorders (Raison & Miller, 2003).

Cortisol also can be used to treat stress disorders.

In an animal model of post-traumatic stress disorder (PTSD), Cohen, Matar, Buskila, Kaplan, and Zohar (2008) looked at giving varying doses of cortisol after a traumatic event. They discovered that a single dose of high dose cortisol immediately after traumatic exposure reduces the prevalence of extreme behavioural disruption. They theorize that the cortisol *"... might disrupt the consolidation of averse or fearful memories."*

In a subject with normally functioning adrenal glands, the level of cortisol goes up after a stressful event. Those with already compromised HPA axis/adrenal glands are the ones that probably cannot mount this vigorous response and therefore suffer the consequences.

This study was done in animals; can the results be applied to humans?

It seems so!

In a pilot study, Aerni et al. (2004) gave low dose cortisol (10mg/day) to three patients with PTSD in a double-blind, placebo-controlled crossover design. The results showed: *"... low dose cortisol treatment reduces the cardinal symptoms of PTSD."*

This was a trial of only three people for three months, so it is not a very powerful trial. Larger studies are needed.

Can PTSD be prevented? Would a dose of cortisol be given to soldiers, trauma victims, rape victims, terrorist victims, victims of crime, prevent PTSD?

There is evidence that this is so.

Schelling, Roozendaal, and De Quervain (2004) showed that *"This protective effect of cortisol can be explained by a cortisol-induced temporary impairment in traumatic memory retrieval which has previously been demonstrated in both rats and humans. Therefore, stress doses of hydrocortisone could be useful for prophylaxis and treatment of PTSD."*

It seems that low dose cortisol can be used to treat PTSD, while a higher dose can be given after a traumatic event to prevent PTSD.

A stressed individual, that is, one with already compromised adrenal glands, will not respond as well to a stressful event as an individual with a normally functioning adrenal glands.

What about other anxieties or phobias?

In the first part of the book, we noted that there are steroid receptors in the brain and that some of these steroids have an action on brain function. Steroids such as DHEA, cortisol and progesterone have been shown to have a positive effect on anxiety and depression (Eser et al., 2006).

I have seen menopausal women suffering anxiety and depression, whose local doctor put them on an anti-depressant. The patients are not happy about this as they feel the depression is more to do with their hormones. When they come off the anti-depressants and start B-HRT, they feel better, their hormone issues are better, and they are no longer anxious or depressed.

Cortisol can be used in the treatment of phobias (Soravia et al., 2006).

Even a single dose of cortisol 40 mg has been shown to reduce anxiety in normal healthy young men (Putman, Hermans, Koppeschaar, van Schijndel, & van Honk, 2007).

However, another study showed that cortisol supplementation did *not* have a profound effect on healthy, non-anxious young men (Soravia, de Quervain, & Heinrichs, 2009). In this study, only a 25 mg cortisol dose was given, while in the previous study, a 40 mg cortisol dose was given, which gave positive results.

A higher dose seems to be more effective.

What about Panic Attacks?

Panic attacks are an episode of intense fear or apprehension that has a sudden onset. The DSM-IV (Diagnostic and Statistical Manual of Mental Disorders 4th revision) describes a panic attack as a discrete period of intense fear or discomfort in which (at least 4 of 13) symptoms listed below, develop abruptly, and reach a peak within ten minutes.

Symptoms include,

- Palpitations, pounding heart, or accelerated heart rate
- Sweating
- Trembling or shaking
- Sensations of shortness of breath or smothering
- Feeling of choking
- Chest pain or discomfort
- Nausea or abdominal distress
- Feeling dizzy, unsteady, lightheaded, or faint
- Feelings of unreality
- Feeling of being detached from oneself
- Fear of losing control or going crazy

- Fear of dying
- Paraesthesia (numbness or tingling sensations)
- Chills or hot flashes

(https://en.wikipedia.org › wiki › Panic_attack
Accessed 6 May 2024)

The combination of symptoms of a racing heart, shaking, and sweating certainly sounds like an adrenaline release and is similar to a 'fight or flight' reaction, although more intense. There may or may not be a precipitating event, although overall the person is generally anxious and stressed. Many think and feel that they are dying. Many feel like they are having a heart attack, call an ambulance and get rushed off to the hospital. They may do this many times, each time being reassured that it is not a heart attack. They keep going because "what if they are really having a heart attack?".

The exact cause is not known, but there are many ideas.

Certainly, cortisol and adrenaline play a part, but other hormones and neurotransmitters, such as gamma amino butyric acid (GABA) and DHEA have also been implicated. GABA is a neurotransmitter and has a role in regulating neuronal excitability. So, you can see why this may be implicated: low GABA = higher neuronal excitability (Goddard et al., 2001).

One of the treatments for anxiety is the use of the class of drugs known as benzodiazepines (diazepam (Valium), oxazepam (Serepax), etc). This class of drugs has been shown to have their effect by stimulating GABA receptors in the brain.

GABA can be supplemented, but the big question is *"Does a GABA supplement pass through the blood-brain barrier (BBB)?"* The research is contradictory (Boonstra et al., 2015).

If GABA does not cross the BBB, how can it work?

Inotsuka, Uchimura, Yamatsu, Kim, and Katakura (2020) suggest that GABA works on the gut and influences the brain via the gut-brain connection.

From a clinical point of view, I personally have seen brilliant responses to a GABA supplement, but then, I have also seen poor or nil response. It is always worth a try.

The other way around this is to boost GABA by supplementing with the amino acid *L-theanine,* which has been shown to elevate GABA levels. This amino acid occurs naturally in green tea, though you would have to drink a lot of green tea to get a reasonable dose.

The dose of L-theanine depends on the individual person and their situation. Research has shown L-theanine to be an extremely safe nutrient. Average dose is 50 to 200mg, although higher doses are possible: the FDA recommends a maximum dose of 1,200 mg.

Still, cups of green tea would help, and it is a pleasant way to relax and reduce stress.

Others have suggested that DHEA may be a factor in panic attacks, especially if there is a low DHEA with normal or high cortisol (excessive DHEA/cortisol ratio). Prolactin is also involved. High prolactin levels have been found during panic attacks.

There is also a suggestion of a familial tendency to panic attacks, so genetics may play a role.

Previous memory and learning and possibly even anticipation also have a role, as anxiety can be something you learn. It could be from a previous stressful event, or just something you have seen on TV. There could also be an element of epigenetics. An anxious pregnant mother can produce an anxious child.

As an example, many people have a fear of snakes or spiders. What would you do if you found a snake in your house? You would more than likely become anxious, you may even panic, or you could have a full-blown panic attack, even though you may never have seen a real snake before.

On the other hand, a snake catcher will be calm and relaxed and possibly even enjoy the situation. This may be an over-the-top example, but hopefully you understand what I am trying to say.

Adrenaline and noradrenaline are also implicated.

Before we go any further, I think it is a good idea to review how the adrenal glands are regulated.

The adrenal glands are not only regulated by ACTH release from the pituitary. If this were the case, then any activation would be too slow to react in an acute situation.

The adrenal glands are also connected to the nervous system so that any stress, real or even perceived, can be acted on immediately.

The nervous system consists of two major parts:

1) the voluntary nervous system, which is the one that we have control over, such as the movement of muscles.

2) the autonomic nervous system (ANS) which largely
we have no control over and controls the vegetative
functions of the body. The ANS consists of two
parts, each having opposite action to each other, the
sympathetic nervous system (SNS) and the para-
sympathetic nervous system (PNS). In health, the
SNS and the PNS are in balance. Like a car, the SNS
is the accelerator, and the PNS is the brake. In balance, both are needed for fine tuning.

At the first sign of stress, and the nature of stress
isn't important - it could be a sabre-tooth tiger or your
tax bill, and even before cortisol is released, parts of the
brain are activated. The SNS is triggered, and this
produces some of the signs of stress due to adrenaline
and noradrenaline release: fast heart rate, sweating, and
so on. The increased SNS also stimulates the adrenal
glands, which release more adrenaline and cortisol.

Note that this SNS activation is virtually an
immediate action. Cortisol is a much slower reaction,
taking hours. If we only relied on cortisol, the sabre-
toothed tiger would have already finished eating you
before cortisol produced any action.

Adrenaline = quick response.

Cortisol = slower, more prolonged, follow-on response.

The SNS also stimulates the hypothalamus to make corticotropin-releasing hormone (CRH) which then stimulates the release of ACTH, which in turn stimulates cortisol release from the adrenal glands. Now there is a feedback loop: cortisol feeds back to suppress the SNS, to reduce noradrenergic activity, as well as to inhibit the CRF and ACTH release.

There is also a relationship between GABA and noradrenaline. Noradrenaline release is mediated, in part through GABA receptors (Sakamaki, Nomura, Yamato, & Tanaka, 2004).

On the other hand, cortisol makes the tissues more sensitive to adrenaline and noradrenaline, so it takes a smaller dose of adrenaline/noradrenaline to elicit a response.

These negative feedback loops are part of the checks and balances to prevent continual cortisol hypersecretion.

In the normal healthy situation, these feedback

loops work in harmony, but something goes wrong in the chronic stress state. The levels of cortisol change, initially they may be elevated, then later with "exhaustion," the levels are lower. Although this is due to HPA axis dysregulation as discussed earlier and not because the adrenal glands "exhaust" themselves.

This influences the adrenaline/noradrenaline system. The ongoing stress continues to activate the SNS and releasing more and more adrenaline and noradrenaline are released. There is heightened tension, and it takes very little to produce a release of hormones that may result in a panic attack. The exact mechanisms are not known and there are many hormones involved; I have tried to give a brief and simple explanation of this very complicated system and to paint a picture of how the body tries to cope with stress, especially when the adrenal glands and the HPA axis have become dysfunctional.

Cortisol has another action: it can activate the enzyme *tryptophan 2, 3, dioxygenase (TDO)* (also known as *tryptophan oxygenase* and/or *tryptophan pyrrolase*). This is a liver enzyme that shunts the amino acid L-tryptophan away from the brain. Therefore, with cortisol activating this enzyme, L-tryptophan levels are reduced, which in turn reduces the level of serotonin in the brain, which was initially thought to lead to depression. The role of serotonin in depression has been

461

disputed recently.

Moncrieff et al. (2023) wrote, *"The main areas of serotonin research provide no consistent evidence of there being an association between serotonin and depression, and no support for the hypothesis that depression is caused by lowered serotonin activity or concentrations."* (Emphasis the author.)

Stress, anxiety, and depression are interrelated and co-exist in many cases. First, there is anxiety, then there is depression. These are largely due to dysfunctional adrenal glands caused by chronic stress. As this is a situation that our species had not encountered before, we therefore have no mechanism to deal with it. The body uses the acute stress response mechanisms repeatedly, but after a time, these mechanisms fail, and the body starts to fall apart.

DHEA

In general, DHEA, or any hormone for that matter, should only be supplemented if:

1) there are symptoms,
2) there is a deficiency, and
3) if the symptoms are consistent with the deficiency.

The guiding principle should be to do a therapeutic trial of physiological replacement.

Earlier, we examined the research into DHEA. From that, it is clear that we do not fully know what DHEA does. We know it is an adrenal hormone, and low levels are associated with many conditions, but we do not know yet how it fits into the scheme of things. We have seen research that shows some improvement in medical conditions if we supplement the missing hormone. We have also seen that the brain does have many DHEA receptors, and that DHEA has an action on brain function.

We will have a closer look at how this all fits into clinical practice.

The first most important thing is we must dismiss the hype that we find on the internet. Words like "super hormone", and "fountain of youth" are bandied about, but what is the truth?

Do we, should we, just give DHEA for one and all?

It is my professional opinion that we should not.

The first thing is to check DHEA levels.

Blood tests are the usual means of doing this. Blood test vs. salivary tests were discussed earlier. A salivary DHEA is included in the baseline adrenal functional test. The routine measurements are cortisol levels at 7.00 am, 12 midday, 6 pm, and 10 pm. DHEA is measured in the 7 am sample.

DHEA is an adrenal hormone; therefore, it is measured as a part of an adrenal assessment. Even a serum DHEA can be regarded as a *de facto* measure of adrenal function.

Symptoms of DHEA deficiency

Symptoms of DHEA deficiency are broad and non-specific and are comparable other hormone deficiencies, especially androgenic. Perhaps the most prominent symptoms are tiredness and fatigue. Others include depression, joint aches and pains, reducing bone and muscle mass, poor libido, dry skin, less axillary hair, difficulty losing weight and poor immunity.

Certainly, if the serum or salivary DHEA is low, then it can be supplemented. When the tests and symptoms indicate a need for supplementation, DHEA can be supplemented on its own but may also be given with other hormones as a part of the overall hormone balance.

However, as a start, it would be a better idea to support the HPA axis and the adrenal glands, diet, nutrition, and lifestyle that reduce stress, before supplementing DHEA.

Causes of low DHEA

As stated earlier, DHEA decreases with age, that is why some have considered it to be the "fountain of youth". The high levels during the younger age can be considered a part of youthfulness, therefore

465

supplementing DHEA will bring back the youth: well, that is the idea anyway!

This does not necessarily work.

Other than ageing, the next most important cause of low DHEA is HPAAD, so the use of DHEA can be part of the treatment. Tiredness, chronic fatigue, and weakness are all symptoms that respond to DHEA.

DHEA is perhaps the most plentiful of steroid hormones and is mildly androgenic, therefore special caution is needed when prescribing for women. The dose should be appropriate, and the levels monitored. In this way, the optimal dose can be discovered.

Again, the principle of supplementation is always to restore levels to normal, not to produce "supermen" or "superwomen". The aim is to provide an improved quality of life.

As the most prominent symptoms are tiredness and fatigue, DHEA can be considered in anyone presenting with these symptoms. Levels must be measured before supplementing.

DHEA has been supplemented in people with chronic fatigue syndrome (CFS) and there has been some success.

Himmel and Seligman (1999) performed a pilot study of white women between ages 35-55 with CFS. The results were quite positive. The study confirmed that a large percentage of people with CFS do have low DHEA levels: in this study 89% of the 116 studied had low DHEA, defined as being less than 2.0 micrograms/ml.

"Supplementation with DHEA to CFS patients lead to a significant reduction in the symptoms of CFS: pain (improved by 18%, p = 0.035), fatigue (decreased by 21%, p = 0.009)), activities of daily living (improved by 8.5%, p = 0.058), helplessness (decreased by 11%, p = 0.015), anxiety (decreased by 35%, p < 0.01), thinking (improved by 26%, p < 0.01), memory (improved by 17%, p < 0.05), and sexual problems (improved by 22%, p = 0.06) over the period of the trial."

Many of the studies done on DHEA make the comment that the results are inconsistent. This is possibly because of inappropriate patient selection. Of course, if you randomly pick 100 people to test DHEA, the results will not be good. However, if appropriate patients were chosen, then results would probably be better. This can be said for *any* trial, testing *any* product, herbal, nutrient, or pharmaceutical.

Cortisol is a catabolic hormone, meaning it breaks down tissue and protein to produce energy. The result is energy, but there is muscle wasting and emaciation. In contrast, DHEA is anabolic, which means it builds up tissue and muscle. In the normal state, the action of cortisol should equal the action of DHEA; all in balance.

The use of DHEA is controversial, especially in mainstream medicine. Certainly, if there is tiredness, fatigue, depression or any other hormonal type of issues, and the levels are low, then DHEA can be, and should be, supplemented.

A good guiding principle is to supplement DHEA as a *therapeutic trial.*

Supplement for two–three months, closely monitor the levels, and frequently review the person. Ask if they are better. Review the symptoms: tiredness, depression, muscle strength and bulk. They will tell you if they are better.

If they say they feel better, then the therapeutic trial was a success, and you should continue.

There are some that say that the DHEA made *no* difference. Then the trial was unsuccessful, so there is no need to continue. This can be said for *all* products: vitamins, minerals nutrients, herbs, bio-identical hormones and even pharmaceuticals.

One definite instance where DHEA supplementation has been shown to be very useful is in the replacement regime in Addison's disease. Conventional doctors do replace cortisol. They also use fludrocortisone acetate, which has an action similar to that of aldosterone, the hormone that controls salt and water balance. What they do not replace is DHEA, yet studies show an improvement in the condition of Addison's disease when this hormone is replaced.

The average oral dose of DHEA is 25-50 mg in women and 50-100 mg in men. In cream form, women can have 1-2% and men 5%, added to their formula.

If the dose is too high in women, they may start to develop some male features such as facial hair growth, deepening of voice, and clitoral enlargement. This generally disappears on reducing the dose. This is one good reason to monitor the person's levels.

There does not seem to be the same "first pass effect" with DHEA as with testosterone, so DHEA can be given orally, although it is even better if it can be incorporated into a cream.

DHEA is not recognised by the mainstream, yet it needs a prescription from a registered general practitioner and needs to be dispensed from a compounding pharmacist.

CONCLUSION

So, what can we conclude from all of this?

First, there is enough evidence to show that the use of synthetic, drug company produced hormones can be dangerous.

Second, there is also enough evidence to demonstrate that the use of the natural, bio-identical hormones is much safer.

Third, the bio-identical hormones are as effective as synthetic hormones.

Fourth, transdermal bio-identical hormones are effective.

Fifth, hormonal issues can be treated without the use of hormone replacement, whether synthetic or natural. Diet, nutrients, herbs, supplements and life-style measures can help these problems.

Sixth, B-HRT replacement is not the first line of

treatment. Depending on the severity of the condition, and unless there are extenuating circumstances, e.g. hysterectomy and oophorectomy, or they have tried everything else, other treatments should be tried first.

Summary

1) Look at the person holistically: treat the person who has symptoms, not just the condition.
2) Exclude other illnesses.
3) Test the hormones.
4) Change diet.
5) Supplement vitamins and minerals.
6) Herbal treatment.
7) Nutrient supplements.
8) Last resort, replace hormones.

Female Hormone Problems

1) Low stress diet.
2) Supplement magnesium, probiotics and St Mary's thistle.
3) Herbs; Vitex, dong quai, maca, black cohosh, fenugreek.
4) Other herbs as needed.
5) Acupuncture
6) B-HRT.

Male Hormone Problems

1) Low stress diet.
2) Improve fitness.
3) Mineral and vitamin supplementation.
4) Herbs; Tribulus, horny goat weed, Tongkat Ali.
5) L-arginine.
6) Acupuncture
7) B-HRT.

HPAAD/Adrenal Exhaustion

1) Low stress diet.
2) Relaxation: meditation, Yoga, Tai Chi, acupuncture.
3) Stress management.
4) Massage, gentle exercise.
5) Adrenal support with herbs, e.g., ashwagandha.
6) Nutrients, especially zinc, vitamin B complex and vitamin C.
7) Phosphatidylserine
8) CRT
9) Supplement DHEA

RECOMMENDED READING

Baratosy, P. (2024). *Death by Civilization*. Peter Baratosy.

Baratosy, P. (2024). *You and Your Gut.* Peter Baratosy.

Baratosy, P. (2023). *The Hypothyroid Syndrome.* Peter Baratosy.

Colborn, T., Dumanoski, D., & Myers, J. P. (1997). *Our Stolen Future*, Penguin Random House: New York, NY.

Jefferies, W. McK. (2004). *Safe Uses of Cortisol* (3rd ed.). Charles C. Thomas: Springfield, IL.

Lee. J. R. & Hopkins, V. (2004). *What Your Doctor May Not Tell You About Menopause: The Breakthrough Book on Hormone Balance* (2nd ed.). Warner Books: New York, NY.

Sapolsky, Robert. (2004). *Why Zebras Don't Get Ulcers* (3rd ed.). Holt Paperbacks: US.

All above books can be ordered online or ordered through any bookshop.

REFERENCES

Abenavoli, L., Capasso, R., Milic, N., & Capasso, F. (2010). Milk thistle in liver diseases: Past, present, future. *Phytother Res, 24*(10), 1423-32. doi: 10.1002/ptr.3207

Adimoelja, A. (2000). Phytochemicals and the breakthrough of traditional herbs in the management of sexual dysfunctions. *Int J Androl, 23* Suppl 2, 82-4. doi: 10.1046/j.1365-2605.2000.00020.x

Aerni, A., Traber, R., Hock, C., Roozendaal, B., Schelling, G., Papassotiropoulos, A., … de Quervain, D. (2004). Low-dose cortisol for symptoms of posttraumatic stress disorder. *Am J Psychiatry, 161*(8), 1488-90. doi: 10.1176/appi.ajp.161.8.1488

Akin, F., Bastemir, M., & Alkis, E. (2007). Effect of insulin sensitivity on SHBG levels in premenopausal versus postmenopausal obese women. *Adv Ther, 24*(6), 1210-20. doi: 10.1007/BF02877767

Akishita, M., Hashimoto, M., Ohike, Y., Ogawa, S., Iijima, K., Eto, M., & Ouchi, Y. (2007). Low testosterone level is an independent determinant of endothelial dysfunction in men. *Hypertens Res, 30*(11), 1029-34. doi: 10.1291/hypres.30.1029

Alexander, C., Cochran, C., Gallicchio, L., Miller, S., Flaws, J., & Zacur, H. (2010). Serum leptin levels, hormone levels, and hot flashes in midlife women. *Fertil Steril, 94*(3):1037-43. doi: 10.1016/j.fertnstert.2009.04.001

Amling, C., Kane, C., Riffenburgh, R., Ward, J., Roberts, J., Lance, R., ... Moul, J. (2001). Relationship between obesity and race in predicting adverse pathologic variables in patients undergoing radical prostatectomy. *Urology, 58*(5), 723-8. doi: 10.1016/s0090-4295(01)01373-5

Anderson, G., Limacher, M., Assaf, A., Bassford, T., Beresford, S., Black, H., ... Wassertheil-Smoller, S (2004). Women's Health Initiative Steering Committee. Effects of conjugated equine estrogen in postmenopausal women with hysterectomy: The Women's Health Initiative randomized controlled trial. *JAMA, 291*(14), 1701-12. doi: 10.1001/jama.291.14.1701

Ang, H, Cheang, H., & Yusof, A. (2000). Effects of Eurycoma longifolia Jack (Tongkat Ali) on the initiation of sexual performance of inexperienced castrated male rats. *Exp Anim, 49*(1), 35-8. doi: 10.1538/expanim.49.35

Ang, H., & Sim, M. (1997). Eurycoma longifolia Jack enhances libido in sexually experienced male rats. *Exp Anim, 46*(4), 287-90. doi: 10.1538/expanim.46.287

Ang, H., Ikeda, S., & Gan, E. (2001). Evaluation of the potency activity of aphrodisiac in Eurycoma longifolia Jack. *Phytother Res, 15*(5), 435-6. doi: 10.1002/ptr.968

Ang, H., Lee, K., & Kiyoshi, M. (2004). Sexual arousal in sexually sluggish old male rats after oral administration of Eurycoma longifolia Jack. *J Basic Clin Physiol Pharmacol, 15*(3-4), 303-9. doi: 10.1515/jbcpp.2004.15.3-4.303

Antonio, J., Uelmen, J., Rodriguez, R., & Earnest, C. (2000). The effects of Tribulus terrestris on body composition and exercise performance in resistance-trained males. *Int J Sport Nutr Exerc Metab, 10*(2), 208-15. doi: 10.1123/ijsnem.10.2.208

Aoki, K., Nakajima, A., Mukasa, K., Osawa, E., Mori, Y., & Sekihara, H. (2003). Prevention of diabetes, hepatic injury, and colon cancer with dehydroepiandrosterone. *J Steroid Biochem Mol Biol,*

85(2-5), 469-72. doi: 10.1016/s0960-0760(03)00219-x

Arlt, W., Callies, F., Koehler, I., van Vlijmen, J., Fassnacht, M., Strasburger, C., … Allolio, B. (2001). Dehydroepiandrosterone supplementation in healthy men with an age-related decline of dehydroepiandrosterone secretion. *J Clin Endocrinol Metab, 86*(10), 4686-92. doi: 10.1210/jcem.86.10.7974

Arslan, A., Koenig, K., Lenner, P., Afanasyeva, Y., Shore, R., Chen, Y., … Zeleniuch-Jacquotte, A. (2014). Circulating estrogen metabolites and risk of breast cancer in postmenopausal women. *Cancer Epidemiol Biomarkers Prev, 23*(7), 1290-7. doi: 10.1158/1055-9965.EPI-14-0009

Auborn, K., Fan, S., Rosen, E., Goodwin, L., Chandraskaren, A., Williams, D., … Carter, T. (2003). Indole-3-carbinol is a negative regulator of estrogen. *J Nutr, 133*(7 Suppl), 2470S-2475S. doi: 10.1093/jn/133.7.2470s

Bailey, T., Cable, N., Aziz, N., Atkinson, G., Cuthbertson, D., Low, D., & Jones, H. (2016). Exercise training reduces the acute physiological severity of post-menopausal hot flushes. *J Physiol, 594*(3), 657-67. doi: 10.1113/JP271456

Bailey, T., Cable, N., Aziz, N., Dobson, R., Sprung, V., Low, D., & Jones, H. (2016). Exercise training reduces the frequency of menopausal hot flushes by improving thermoregulatory control. *Menopause, 23*(7), 708-18. doi: 10.1097/GME.0000000000000625

Bailly, C. (2021). Medicinal properties and anti-inflammatory components of Phytolacca (Shenglu). *Digital Chinese Medicine, 4*(3), 159-169. doi: 10.1016/j.dcmed.2021.09.001

Balazs, Z., Schweizer, R., Frey, F., Rohner-Jeanrenaud, F., & Odermatt, A. (2008). DHEA induces 11 -HSD2 by acting on CCAAT/enhancer-binding proteins. *J Am Soc Nephrol, 19*(1), 92-101. doi: 10.1681/ASN.2007030263

Band, P., Deschamps, M., Falardeau, M., Ladouceur, J., & Cote, J. (1984). Treatment of benign breast disease with vitamin A. *Prev Med, 13*(5), 549-54. doi: 10.1016/0091-7435(84)90023-9

Bános, C., Takó, J., Salamon, F., Györgyi, S., & Czikkely, R. (1979). Effect of ACTH-stimulated glucocorticoid hypersecretion on the serum concentrations of thyroxine-binding globulin, thyroxine, triiodothyronine, reverse triiodothyronine and on the TSH-response to TRH. *Acta Med Acad Sci Hung, 36*(4), 381-94

Baschetti R. (2003). Chronic fatigue syndrome: An endocrine disease off limits for endocrinologists? *Eur J Clin Invest, 33*(12),1029-31. doi: 10.1111/j.1365-2362.2003.01272.x

Baulieu, E., Thomas, G., Legrain, S., Lahlou, N., Roger, M., Debuire, B., … Forette, F. (2000). Dehydroepiandrosterone (DHEA), DHEA sulfate, and aging: Contribution of the DHEAge Study to a sociobiomedical issue. *Proc Natl Acad Sci U S A, 97*(8), 4279-84. doi: 10.1073/pnas.97.8.4279

Beezhold, B., Radnitz, C., McGrath, R., & Feldman, A. (2018). Vegans report less bothersome vasomotor and physical menopausal symptoms than omnivores. *Maturitas, 112*, 12-17. doi: 10.1016/j.maturitas.2018.03.009

Bélanger, A., Locong, A., Noel, C., Cusan, L., Dupont, A., Prévost, J., … Sévigny, J. (1989). Influence of diet on plasma steroids and sex hormone-binding globulin levels in adult men. *J Steroid Biochem, 32*(6), 829-33. doi: 10.1016/0022-4731(89)90459-7

Beral V; Million Women Study Collaborators. (2003). Breast cancer and hormone-replacement therapy in the Million Women Study. *Lancet, 362*(9382), 419-27. doi: 10.1016/s0140-6736(03)14065-2

Berrino, F., Bellati, C., Secreto, G., Camerini, E., Pala, V., Panico, S., ... Kaaks, R. (2001). Reducing bioavailable sex hormones through a comprehensive change in diet: The diet and androgens (DIANA) randomized trial. *Cancer Epidemiol Biomarkers Prev, 10*(1), 25-33.

Bhatia, B., & Price, C. (2001). Insulin alters the effects of follicle-stimulating hormone on aromatase in bovine granulosa cells in vitro. *Steroids, 66*(6), 511-9. doi: 10.1016/s0039-128x(00)00218-x

Billups, K., Bank, A., Padma-Nathan, H., Katz, S., & Williams, R. (2005). Erectile dysfunction is a marker for cardiovascular disease: Results of the minority health institute expert advisory panel. *J Sex Med, 2*(1), 40-50; discussion 50-2. doi: 10.1111/j.1743-6109.2005.20104_1.x

Birks, J., & Harvey, R. (2018). Donepezil for dementia due to Alzheimer's disease. *Cochrane Database Syst Rev, 6*(6), CD001190. doi: 10.1002/14651858.CD001190.pub3

Bitzer, J., Kenemans, P., & Mueck, A. (2008). FSDeducation Group. Breast cancer risk in postmenopausal women using testosterone in combination with hormone replacement therapy. *Maturitas, 59*(3), 209-18. doi:

10.1016/j.maturitas.2008.01.005

Blatt, J., Van Le, L., Weiner, T., & Sailer, S. (2003). Ovarian carcinoma in an adolescent with transgenerational exposure to diethylstilbestrol. *J Pediatr Hematol Oncol, 25*(8), 635-6. doi: 10.1097/00043426-200308000-00009

Bloch, M., Schmidt, P., Danaceau, M., Adams, L., & Rubinow, D. (1999). Dehydroepiandrosterone treatment of midlife dysthymia. *Biol Psychiatry, 45*(12), 1533-41. doi: 10.1016/s0006-3223(99)00066-9

Boonstra, E., de Kleijn, R., Colzato, L., Alkemade, A., Forstmann, B., & Nieuwenhuis, S. (2015). Neurotransmitters as food supplements: The effects of GABA on brain and behavior. *Front Psychol, 6*, 1520. doi: 10.3389/fpsyg.2015.01520

Bortz, W. 2nd., & Wallace, D. (1999). Physical fitness, aging, and sexuality. *West J Med, 170*(3), 167-9.

Botwood, N., Hamilton-Fairley, D., Kiddy, D., Robinson, S., & Franks, S. (1995). Sex hormone-binding globulin and female reproductive function. *J Steroid Biochem Mol Biol, 53*(1-6), 529-31. doi: 10.1016/0960-0760(95)00108-c

Bower, W., Johns, M., Margolis, H., Williams, I., & Bell, B. (2007). Population-based surveillance for acute liver failure. *Am J Gastroenterol, 102*(11), 2459-63. doi: 10.1111/j.1572-0241.2007.01388.x

Brandão-Neto, J., de Mendonça, B., Shuhama, T., Marchini, J., Pimenta, W., & Tornero, M. (1990). Zinc acutely and temporarily inhibits adrenal cortisol secretion in humans. A preliminary report. *Biol Trace Elem Res, 24*(1), 83-9. doi: 10.1007/BF02789143

Breu, W., Hagenlocher, M., Redl, K., Tittel, G., Stadler, F., & Wagner, H. (1992). Antiphlogistische Wirkung eines mit hyperkritischem Kohlendioxid gewonnenen Sabalfrucht-Extraktes. In-vitro-Hemmung des Cyclooxygenase- und 5-Lipoxygenase-Metabolismus [Anti-inflammatory activity of sabal fruit extracts prepared with supercritical carbon dioxide. In vitro antagonists of cyclooxygenase and 5-lipoxygenase metabolism]. *Arzneimittelforschung, 42*(4), 547-51. German.

Brinton, R., Thompson, R., Foy, M., Baudry, M., Wang, J., Finch, C., … Nilsen, J. (2008). Progesterone receptors: Form and function in brain. *Front Neuroendocrinol, 29*(2), 313-39. doi: 10.1016/j.yfrne.2008.02.001

Brown, R., Cascio, C., & Papadopoulos, V. (2000). Pathways of neurosteroid biosynthesis in cell lines from human brain: Regulation of dehydroepiandrosterone formation by oxidative stress and beta-amyloid peptide. *J Neurochem, 74*(2), 847-59. doi: 10.1046/j.1471-4159.2000.740847.x

Bu, S., Yin, D., Ren, X., Jiang, L., Wu, Z., Gao, Q., & Pei, G. (1997). Progesterone induces apoptosis and up-regulation of p53 expression in human ovarian carcinoma cell lines. *Cancer, 79*(10), 1944-50. doi: 10.1002/(sici)1097-0142(19970515)79:10<1944:aid-cncr15>3.0.co;2-v

Buckley, N., & Eddleston, M. (2005). Paracetamol (acetaminophen) poisoning. *Clin Evid,* (14), 1738-44.

Burry, K., Patton, P., & Hermsmeyer, K. (1999). Percutaneous absorption of progesterone in postmenopausal women treated with transdermal estrogen. *Am J Obstet Gynecol, 180*(6 Pt 1), 1504-11. doi: 10.1016/s0002-9378(99)70046-3

Bury, N., Chung, M., Sturm, A., Walker, P., & Hogstrand, C. (2008). Cortisol stimulates the zinc signaling pathway and expression of metallothioneins and ZnT1 in rainbow trout gill epithelial cells. *Am J Physiol Regul Integr Comp Physiol, 294*(2), R623-9. doi: 10.1152/ajpregu.00646.2007

Cabeza, M., Bratoeff, E., Heuze, I., Rojas, A., Terán, N., Ochoa, M., ... Gracia, I. (2006). New progesterone derivatives as inhibitors of 5alpha-reductase enzyme and prostate cancer cell growth. *J Enzyme Inhib Med Chem, 21*(4), 371-8. doi: 10.1080/14756360600748474

Cadegiani, F., & Kater, C. (2016). Adrenal fatigue does not exist: A systematic review. *BMC Endocr Disord, 16*(1), 48. doi: 10.1186/s12902-016-0128-4.

Campbell, D., & Kurzer, M. (1993). Flavonoid inhibition of aromatase enzyme activity in human preadipocytes. *J Steroid Biochem Mol Biol, 46*(3), 381-8. doi: 10.1016/0960-0760(93)90228-o

Carroll, J., Rosario, E., Chang, L., Stanczyk, F., Oddo, S., LaFerla, F., & Pike, C. (2007). Progesterone and estrogen regulate Alzheimer-like neuropathology in female 3xTg-AD mice. *J Neurosci, 27*(48), 13357-65. doi: 10.1523/JNEUROSCI.2718-07.2007

Cayan, F., Tek, M., Balli, E., Oztuna, S., Karazindiyanoğlu, S., & Cayan, S. (2008). The effect of testosterone alone and testosterone + estradiol therapy on bladder functions and smooth muscle/collagen content in surgically menopause induced rats. *Maturitas, 60*(3-4), 248-52. doi: 10.1016/j.maturitas.2008.07.008

Chan, W., Carrell, R., Zhou, A., & Read, R. (2013). How changes in affinity of corticosteroid-binding globulin modulate free cortisol concentration. *J Clin Endocrinol Metab, 98*(8), 3315-22. doi: 10.1210/jc.2012-4280

Chan, W., Carrell, R., Zhou, A., & Read, R. (2013). How changes in affinity of corticosteroid-binding globulin modulate free cortisol concentration. *J Clin Endocrinol Metab*, *98*(8), 3315-22. doi: 10.1210/jc.2012-4280

Chang, K., Lee, T., Linares-Cruz, G., Fournier, S., & de Ligniéres, B. (1995). Influences of percutaneous administration of estradiol and progesterone on human breast epithelial cell cycle in vivo. *Fertil Steril, 63*(4), 785-91.

Chattha, R., Raghuram, N., Venkatram, P., & Hongasandra, N. (2008). Treating the climacteric symptoms in Indian women with an integrated approach to yoga therapy: A randomized control study. *Menopause, 15*(5), 862-70. doi: 10.1097/gme.0b013e318167b902

Chedrawe, E., Sathe, A., White, J., Ory, J., & Ramasamy, R. (2022). Testosterone therapy in advanced prostate cancer. *Androg Clin Res Ther, 3*(1), 180-186. doi: 10.1089/andro.2021.0035

Chen, T., & Holick, M. (2003). Vitamin D and prostate cancer prevention and treatment. *Trends Endocrinol Metab, 14*(9), 423-30. doi: 10.1016/j.tem.2003.09.004

Chen, C., Gong, X., Yang, X., Shang, X., Du, Q., Liao, Q., ... Xu, J. (2019). The roles of estrogen and estrogen receptors in gastrointestinal disease. *Oncol Lett, 18*(6), 5673-5680. doi: 10.3892/ol.2019.10983

Chen, J., Wollman, Y., Chernichovsky, T., Iaina, A., Sofer, M., & Matzkin, H. (1999). Effect of oral administration of high-dose nitric oxide donor L-arginine in men with organic erectile dysfunction: Results of a double-blind, randomized, placebo-controlled study. *BJU Int, 83*(3), 269-73. doi: 10.1046/j.1464-410x.1999.00906.x

Chen, R., Yu, Y., & Dong, X. (2017). Progesterone receptor in the prostate: A potential suppressor for benign prostatic hyperplasia and prostate cancer. *J Steroid Biochem Mol Biol, 166*:91-96. doi: 10.1016/j.jsbmb.2016.04.008

Chen, S. (2002). Modulation of aromatase activity and expression by environmental chemicals. *Front Biosci, 7*, d1712-9. doi: 10.2741/a874

Chen, W., Zhou, X., Chen, D., & Kang, J. (1988). Effects of cimetidine, progesterone, cannitracin and tolazoline on the weight and DNA content of the testosterone-induced hyperplastic prostate of the rat. *Urol Res, 16*(5), 363-6. doi: 10.1007/BF00256043

Chopra, I. (1977). A study of extrathyroidal conversion of thyroxine (T4) to 3,3',5-triiodothyronine (T3) in vitro. *Endocrinology, 101*(2), 453-63. doi: 10.1210/endo-101-2-453

Cleare, A., Heap, E., Malhi, G., Wessely, S., O'Keane, V., & Miell, J. (1999). Low-dose hydrocortisone in chronic fatigue syndrome: A randomised crossover trial. *Lancet, 353*(9151), 455-8. doi: 10.1016/S0140-6736(98)04074-4

Cleare, A., Miell, J., Heap, E., Sookdeo, S., Young, L., Malhi, G., & O'Keane, V. (2001). Hypothalamo-pituitary-adrenal axis dysfunction in chronic fatigue syndrome, and the effects of low-dose hydrocortisone therapy. *J Clin Endocrinol Metab, 86*(8), 3545-54. doi: 10.1210/jcem.86.8.7735

Cochran, C., Gallicchio, L., Miller, S., Zacur, H., & Flaws, J. (2008). Cigarette smoking, androgen levels, and hot flushes in midlife women. *Obstet Gynecol, 112*(5), 1037-44. doi: 10.1097/AOG.0b013e318189a8e2

Cohen, H., Matar, M., Buskila, D., Kaplan, Z., & Zohar, J. (2008). Early post-stressor intervention with high-dose corticosterone attenuates posttraumatic stress response in an animal model of posttraumatic stress disorder. *Biol Psychiatry, 64*(8), 708-717. doi: 10.1016/j.biopsych.2008.05.025

Cohen, S., Janicki-Deverts, D., Doyle, W., Miller, G., Frank, E., Rabin, B., & Turner, R. (2012). Chronic stress, glucocorticoid receptor resistance, inflammation, and disease risk. *Proc Natl Acad Sci U S A, 109*(16), 5995-9. doi: 10.1073/pnas.1118355109

Cohen, S., Janicki-Deverts, D., Doyle, W., Miller, G., Frank, E., Rabin, B., & Turner, R. (2012). Chronic stress, glucocorticoid receptor resistance, inflammation, and disease risk. *Proc Natl Acad Sci U S A, 109*(16), 5995-9. doi: 10.1073/pnas.1118355109

Colborn, T., Dumanoski, D., & Myers, J. (1996). *Our Stolen Future.* Abacus Books.

Colditz, G., Hankinson, S., Hunter, D., Willett, W., Manson, J., Stampfer, M., ... Speizer, F. (1995). The use of estrogens and progestins and the risk of breast cancer in postmenopausal women. *N Engl J Med, 332*(24), 1589-93. doi: 10.1056/NEJM199506153322401

Courtney, C., Farrell, D., Gray, R., Hills, R., Lynch, L., Sellwood, E., ... Bentham, P. (2004). AD2000 Collaborative Group. Long-term donepezil treatment in 565 patients with Alzheimer's disease (AD2000):

Randomised double-blind trial. *Lancet, 363*(9427), 2105-15. doi: 10.1016/S0140-6736(04)16499-4

D'Andrea, A., Caso, P., Salerno, G., Scarafile, R., De Corato, G., Mita, C., ... Calabrò, R. (2007). Left ventricular early myocardial dysfunction after chronic misuse of anabolic-androgenic steroids: A doppler myocardial and strain imaging analysis. *Br J Sports Med, 41*(3), 149-55. doi: 10.1136/bjsm.2006.030171

Darbre, P., & Charles, A. (2010). Environmental oestrogens and breast cancer: Evidence for combined involvement of dietary, household and cosmetic xenoestrogens. *Anticancer Res, 30*(3), 815-27.

Davey Smith, G., Frankel, S., & Yarnell, J. (1997). Sex and death: Are they related? Findings from the Caerphilly Cohort Study. *BMJ, 315*(7123), 1641-4. doi: 10.1136/bmj.315.7123.1641

Davis, S. (1999). Androgen treatment in women. *Med J Aust, 170*(11), 545-9.

Davis, S., McCloud, P., Strauss, B., & Burger, H. (1995). Testosterone enhances estradiol's effects on postmenopausal bone density and sexuality. *Maturitas, 21*(3), 227-36. doi: 10.1016/0378-5122(94)00898-h

Davis, S., Moreau, M., Kroll, R., Bouchard, C., Panay, N., Gass, M., ... Studd, J. (2008). APHRODITE Study

Team. Testosterone for low libido in postmenopausal women not taking estrogen. *N Engl J Med, 359*(19), 2005-17. doi: 10.1056/NEJMoa0707302

de Lignieres, B. (1993). Transdermal dihydrotestosterone treatment of 'andropause'. *Ann Med, 25*(3), 235-41. doi: 10.3109/07853899309147869

de Lignières, B. (2002). Effects of progestogens on the postmenopausal breast. *Climacteric, 5*(3), 229-35. doi: 10.1080/713605271

Debing, E., Peeters, E., Duquet, W., Poppe, K., Velkeniers, B., & Van den Brande, P. (2007). Endogenous sex hormone levels in postmenopausal women undergoing carotid artery endarterectomy. *Eur J Endocrinol, 156*(6), 687-93. doi: 10.1530/EJE-06-0702

Debing, E., Peeters, E., Duquet, W., Poppe, K., Velkeniers, B., & Van Den Brande, P. (2008). Men with atherosclerotic stenosis of the carotid artery have lower testosterone levels compared with controls. *Int Angiol, 27*(2), 135-41.

Deenadayalu, V., White, R., Stallone, J., Gao, X., & Garcia, A. (2001). Testosterone relaxes coronary arteries by opening the large-conductance, calcium-activated potassium channel. *Am J Physiol Heart Circ Physiol, 281*(4), H1720-7. doi: 10.1152/ajpheart.2001.281.4.H1720

Dell'Agli, M., Galli, G., Dal Cero, E., Belluti, F., Matera, R., Zironi. E., ... Bosisio, E. (2008). Potent inhibition of human phosphodiesterase-5 by icariin derivatives. *J Nat Prod, 71*(9), 1513-7. doi: 10.1021/np800049y

Dennerstein, L., Smith, A., Morse, C., Burger, H., Green, A., Hopper, J., & Ryan, M. (1993). Menopausal symptoms in Australian women. *Med J Aust, 159*(4), 232-6. doi: 10.5694/j.1326-5377.1993.tb137821.x

Derby, C, Mohr, B., Goldstein, I., Feldman, H., Johannes, C., & McKinlay, J. (2000). Modifiable risk factors and erectile dysfunction: Can lifestyle changes modify risk? *Urology, 56*(2), 302-6. doi: 10.1016/s0090-4295(00)00614-2

Di Monaco, M., Pizzini, A., Gatto, V., Leonardi, L., Gallo, M., Brignardello, E., & Boccuzzi, G. (1997). Role of glucose-6-phosphate dehydrogenase inhibition in the antiproliferative effects of dehydroepiandrosterone on human breast cancer cells. *Br J Cancer, 75*(4), 589-92. doi: 10.1038/bjc.1997.102

Dickerman, R., Schaller, F., Zachariah, N., & McConathy, W. (1997). Left ventricular size and function in elite bodybuilders using anabolic steroids. *Clin J Sport Med, 7*(2), 90-3. doi: 10.1097/00042752-199704000-00003

Dickerman, R., Schaller, F., & McConathy, W. (1998). Left ventricular wall thickening does occur in elite power athletes with or without anabolic steroid Use. *Cardiology, 90*(2), 145-8. doi: 10.1159/000006834

Dimitrakakis, C., Jones, R., Liu, A., & Bondy, C. (2004). Breast cancer incidence in postmenopausal women using testosterone in addition to usual hormone therapy. *Menopause, 11*(5), 531-5. doi: 10.1097/01.gme.0000119983.48235.d3

Dormire, S., & Howharn, C. (2007). The effect of dietary intake on hot flashes in menopausal women. *J Obstet Gynecol Neonatal Nurs, 36*(3), 255-62. doi: 10.1111/j.1552-6909.2007.00142.x

Dormire, S., & Reame, N. (2003). Menopausal hot flash frequency changes in response to experimental manipulation of blood glucose. *Nurs Res, 52*(5), 338-43. doi: 10.1097/00006199-200309000-00008

Ducrey, B., Marston, A., Göhring, S., Hartmann, R., & Hostettmann, K. (1997). Inhibition of 5 alpha-reductase and aromatase by the ellagitannins oenothein A and oenothein B from Epilobium species. *Planta Med, 63*(2), 111-4. doi: 10.1055/s-2006-957624

Dutta, S., Banu, S., & Arosh, J. (2023). Endocrine disruptors and endometriosis. *Reprod Toxicol, 115*, 56-73. doi: 10.1016/j.reprotox.2022.11.007

Ebrahim, S., May, M., Ben Shlomo, Y., McCarron, P., Frankel, S., Yarnell, J., & Davey Smith, G. (2002). Sexual intercourse and risk of ischaemic stroke and coronary heart disease: the Caerphilly study. *J Epidemiol Community Health, 56*(2), 99-102. doi: 10.1136/jech.56.2.99

Eliassen, A., Missmer, S., Tworoger, S., & Hankinson, S. (2008). Circulating 2-hydroxy- and 16alpha-hydroxy estrone levels and risk of breast cancer among postmenopausal women. *Cancer Epidemiol Biomarkers Prev, 17*(8), 2029-35. doi: 10.1158/1055-9965.EPI-08-0262

el-Sheikh, M., Dakkak, M., & Saddique, A. (1988). The effect of Permixon on androgen receptors. *Acta Obstet Gynecol Scand, 67*(5), 397-9. doi: 10.3109/00016348809004247

English, K., Steeds, R., Jones, T., Diver, M., & Channer, K. (2000). Low-dose transdermal testosterone therapy improves angina threshold in men with chronic stable angina: A randomized, double-blind, placebo-controlled study. *Circulation, 102*(16), 1906-11. doi: 10.1161/01.cir.102.16.1906

Eser, D., Romeo, E., Baghai, T., Schüle, C., Zwanzger, P., & Rupprecht, R. (2006). Neuroactive steroids as modulators of depression and anxiety. *Expert Rev*

Endocrinol Metab, 1(4), 517-526. doi:
10.1586/17446651.1.4.517

Fabre, A., Fournier, A., Mesrine, S., Gompel, A.,
Desreux, J., Berrino, F., ... Clavel-Chapelon, F. (2008).
Progestagens use before menopause and breast cancer
risk according to histology and hormone receptors.
Cancer Epidemiol Biomarkers Prev, 17(10), 2723-8.
doi: 10.1158/1055-9965.EPI-08-0056

Fanzo, J., Reaves, S., Cui, L., Zhu, L., Wu, J., Wang, Y.,
& Lei, K. (2001). Zinc status affects p53, gadd45, and
c-fos expression and caspase-3 activity in human
bronchial epithelial cells. *Am J Physiol Cell Physiol,
281*(3), C751-7. doi: 10.1152/ajpcell.2001.281.3.C751

Farnsworth, W. (1996). Roles of estrogen and SHBG in
prostate physiology. *Prostate, 28*(1), 17-23. doi:
10.1002/(SICI)1097-0045(199601)28:1<17:AID-
PROS3>3.0.CO;2-L

Faure, E., Chantre, P., & Mares, P. (2002). Effects of a
standardized soy extract on hot flushes: A multicenter,
double-blind, randomized, placebo-controlled study.
Menopause, 9(5), 329-34. doi: 10.1097/00042192-
200209000-00005

Fisher, A., Bandini, E., Rastrelli, G., Corona, G.,
Monami, M., Mannucci, E., & Maggi, M. (2012).
Sexual and cardiovascular correlates of male
497

unfaithfulness. *J Sex Med, 9*(6), 1508-18. doi:
10.1111/j.1743-6109.2012.02722.x

Fitzpatrick, M. (2005). Selling sickness: How drug
companies are turning us all into patients. *BMJ,
331*(7518), 701.

Flynn, M., Weaver-Osterholtz, D., Sharpe-Timms, K.,
Allen, S., & Krause, G. (1999).
Dehydroepiandrosterone replacement in aging humans.
J Clin Endocrinol Metab, 84(5), 1527-33. doi:
10.1210/jcem.84.5.5672

Formby, B., & Wiley, T. (1998). Progesterone inhibits
growth and induces apoptosis in breast cancer cells:
Inverse effects on Bcl-2 and p53. *Ann Clin Lab Sci,
28*(6), 360-9.

Fournier, A., Berrino, F., & Clavel-Chapelon, F. (2008).
Unequal risks for breast cancer associated with
different hormone replacement therapies: Results from
the E3N cohort study. *Breast Cancer Res Treat, 107*(1),
103-11. doi: 10.1007/s10549-007-9523-x

Fournier, A., Berrino, F., Riboli, E., Avenel, V., &
Clavel-Chapelon, F. (2005). Breast cancer risk in
relation to different types of hormone replacement
therapy in the E3N-EPIC cohort. *Int J Cancer, 114*(3),
448-54. doi: 10.1002/ijc.20710

Fournier, A., Mesrine, S., Boutron-Ruault, M., & Clavel-Chapelon, F. (2009). Estrogen-progestagen menopausal hormone therapy and breast cancer: Does delay from menopause onset to treatment initiation influence risks? *J Clin Oncol, 27*(31), 5138-43. doi: 10.1200/JCO.2008.21.6432

Freedman, R. (2002). Core body temperature variation in symptomatic and asymptomatic postmenopausal women: Brief report. *Menopause, 9*(6), 399-401. doi: 10.1097/00042192-200211000-00004

Freedman, R. (2014). Menopausal hot flashes: Mechanisms, endocrinology, treatment. *J Steroid Biochem Mol Biol, 142*, 115-20. doi: 10.1016/j.jsbmb.2013.08.010

Freedman, R., Norton, D., Woodward, S., & Cornélissen, G. (1995). Core body temperature and circadian rhythm of hot flashes in menopausal women. *J Clin Endocrinol Metab, 80*(8), 2354-8. doi: 10.1210/jcem.80.8.7629229

Fuller, S., Tan, R., & Martins, R. (2007). Androgens in the etiology of Alzheimer's disease in aging men and possible therapeutic interventions. *J Alzheimers Dis, 12*(2), 129-42. doi: 10.3233/jad-2007-12202

Galiè, N., Brundage, B., Ghofrani, H., Oudiz, R., Simonneau, G., Safdar, Z., … Barst, R. (2009).

Pulmonary Arterial Hypertension and Response to Tadalafil (PHIRST) Study Group.Tadalafil therapy for pulmonary arterial hypertension. *Circulation, 119*(22), 2894-903. doi: 10.1161/CIRCULATIONAHA.108.839274

GamalEl Din, S., Abdel Salam, M., Mohamed, M., Ahmed, A., Motawaa, A., Saadeldin, O., & Elnabarway, R. (2019). Tribulus terrestris versus placebo in the treatment of erectile dysfunction and lower urinary tract symptoms in patients with late-onset hypogonadism: A placebo-controlled study. *Urologia, 86*(2), 74-78. doi: 10.1177/0391560318802160

Gauthaman, K., & Ganesan, A. (2008). The hormonal effects of Tribulus terrestris and its role in the management of male erectile dysfunction—an evaluation using primates, rabbit and rat. *Phytomedicine, 15*(1-2), 44-54. doi: 10.1016/j.phymed.2007.11.011

Gauthaman, K., Adaikan, P., & Prasad, R. (2002). Aphrodisiac properties of Tribulus Terrestris extract (Protodioscin) in normal and castrated rats. *Life Sci, 71*(12), 1385-96. doi: 10.1016/s0024-3205(02)01858-1

George, M., Guidotti, A., Rubinow, D., Pan, B., Mikalauskas, K., & Post, R. (1994). CSF neuroactive steroids in affective disorders: pregnenolone, progesterone, and DBI. *Biol Psychiatry, 35*(10), 775-80. doi: 10.1016/0006-3223(94)91139-8

Ghent, W., Eskin, B., Low, D., & Hill, L. (1993). Iodine replacement in fibrocystic disease of the breast. *Can J Surg, 36*(5), 453-60.

Giovannucci, E. (1999). Tomatoes, tomato-based products, lycopene, and cancer: Review of the epidemiologic literature. *J Natl Cancer Inst, 91*(4), 317-31. doi: 10.1093/jnci/91.4.317

Giovannucci, E., Ascherio, A., Rimm, E., Stampfer, M., Colditz, G., & Willett, W. (1995). Intake of carotenoids and retinol in relation to risk of prostate cancer. *J Natl Cancer Inst, 87*(23), 1767-76. doi: 10.1093/jnci/87.23.1767

Giovannucci, E., Rimm, E., Liu, Y., Stampfer, M., & Willett, W. (2002). A prospective study of tomato products, lycopene, and prostate cancer risk. *J Natl Cancer Inst, 94*(5), 391-8. doi: 10.1093/jnci/94.5.391

Goddard, A., Mason, G., Almai, A., Rothman, D., Behar, K., Petroff, O., ... Krystal, J. (2001). Reductions in occipital cortex GABA levels in panic disorder detected with 1h-magnetic resonance spectroscopy. *Arch Gen Psychiatry, 58*(6), 556-61. doi: 10.1001/archpsyc.58.6.556

Gordon, P., Kerwin, J., Boesen, K., & Senf, J. (2006). Sertraline to treat hot flashes: A randomized controlled, double-blind, crossover trial in a general population. *Menopause, 13*(4), 568-75. doi: 10.1097/01.gme.0000196595.82452.ca

Gotmar, A., Hammar, M., Fredrikson, M., Samsioe, G., Nerbrand, C., Lidfeldt, J., & Spetz, A. (2008). Symptoms in peri- and postmenopausal women in relation to testosterone concentrations: Data from The Women's Health in the Lund Area (WHILA) study. *Climacteric, 11*(4), 304-14. doi: 10.1080/13697130802249769

Grady, D., Cohen, B., Tice, J., Kristof, M., Olyaie, A., & Sawaya, G. (2007). Ineffectiveness of sertraline for treatment of menopausal hot flushes: A randomized controlled trial. *Obstet Gynecol, 109*(4), 823-30. doi: 10.1097/01.AOG.0000258278.73505.fa

Graham, M., Grace, F., Boobier, W., Hullin, D., Kicman, A., Cowan, D., ... Baker, J. (2006). Homocysteine induced cardiovascular events: A consequence of long term anabolic-androgenic steroid (AAS) abuse. *Br J Sports Med, 40*(7), 644-8. doi: 10.1136/bjsm.2005.025668

Gröschl, M. (2008). Current status of salivary hormone analysis. *Clin Chem, 54*(11), 1759-69. doi:

10.1373/clinchem.2008.108910

Gurnell, E., Hunt, P., Curran, S., Conway, C., Pullenayegum, E., Huppert, F., ... Chatterjee, V. (2008). Long-term DHEA replacement in primary adrenal insufficiency: A randomized, controlled trial. *J Clin Endocrinol Metab, 93*(2), 400-9. doi: 10.1210/jc.2007-1134

Habito, R., & Ball, M. (2001). Postprandial changes in sex hormones after meals of different composition. *Metabolism, 50*(5), 505-11. doi: 10.1053/meta.2001.20973

Hackney, A., Feith, S., Pozos, R., & Seale, J. (1995). Effects of high altitude and cold exposure on resting thyroid hormone concentrations. *Aviat Space Environ Med, 66*(4), 325-9.

Hajjar, R., Kaiser, F., & Morley, J. (1997). Outcomes of long-term testosterone replacement in older hypogonadal males: A retrospective analysis. *J Clin Endocrinol Metab, 82*(11), 3793-6. doi: 10.1210/jcem.82.11.4387

Hall, S., Shackelton, R., Rosen, R., & Araujo, A. (2010). Sexual activity, erectile dysfunction, and incident cardiovascular events. *Am J Cardiol, 105*(2), 192-7. doi: 10.1016/j.amjcard.2009.08.671

Hamzah, S., & Yusof, A. (2003). The ergogenic effects of Eurycoma longifolia Jack: A pilot study. *Br J Sports Med*, *37*, 464-470.

Hartgens, F., & Kuipers, H. (2004). Effects of androgenic-anabolic steroids in athletes. *Sports Med*, *34*(8), 513-54. doi: 10.2165/00007256-200434080-00003

Hassan, S., Thacharodi, A., Priya, A., Meenatchi, R., Hegde, T., Thangamani, R., ... Pugazhendhi, A. (2024). Endocrine disruptors: Unravelling the link between chemical exposure and Women's reproductive health. *Environ Res*, *241*, 117385. doi: 10.1016/j.envres.2023.117385

Hellhammer, J., Fries, E., Buss, C., Engert, V., Touch, A., Rutenberg, D., & Hellhammer, D. (2004). Effects of soy lecithin phosphatidic acid and phosphatidylserine complex (PAS) on the endocrine and psychological responses to mental stress. *Stress*, *7*(2), 119-26. doi: 10.1080/10253890410001728379

Henderson, E., Weinberg, M., & Wright, W. (1950). Pregnenolone. *J Clin Endocrinol Metab*, *10*(4), 455-74. doi: 10.1210/jcem-10-4-455

Henderson, V., Paganini-Hill, A., Miller, B., Elble, R., Reyes, P., Shoupe, D., ... Farlow, M. (2000). Estrogen for Alzheimer's disease in women: Randomized, double-blind, placebo-controlled trial. *Neurology, 54*(2), 295-301. doi: 10.1212/wnl.54.2.295

Hendrix, S., Cochrane, B., Nygaard, I., Handa, V., Barnabei, V., Iglesia, C., ... McNeeley, S. (2005). Effects of estrogen with and without progestin on urinary incontinence. *JAMA, 293*(8), 935-48. doi: 10.1001/jama.293.8.935

Hermann, A., Nafziger, A., Victory, J., Kulawy, R., Rocci, M. Jr., & Bertino, J. Jr. (2005). Over-the-counter progesterone cream produces significant drug exposure compared to a food and drug administration-approved oral progesterone product. *J Clin Pharmacol, 45*(6), 614-9. doi: 10.1177/0091270005276621

Hermsmeyer, R., Thompson, T., Pohost, G., & Kaski, J. (2008). Cardiovascular effects of medroxyprogesterone acetate and progesterone: A case of mistaken identity? *Nat Clin Pract Cardiovasc Med, 5*(7), 387-95. doi: 10.1038/ncpcardio1234

Heydari, B., & Le Mellédo, J. (2002). Low pregnenolone sulphate plasma concentrations in patients with generalized social phobia. *Psychol Med, 32*(5), 929-33. doi: 10.1017/s0033291702005238

Himmel, P., & Seligman, T. (1999). A pilot study employing dehydroepiandrosterone (DHEA) in the treatment of chronic fatigue syndrome. *J Clin*

Rheumatol, 5(2), 56-9. doi: 10.1097/00124743-199904000-00004

Hirano, T., Homma, M., & Oka, K. (1994). Effects of stinging nettle root extracts and their steroidal components on the Na+, K(+)-ATPase of the benign prostatic hyperplasia. *Planta Med, 60*(1), 30-3. doi: 10.1055/s-2006-959402

Hirst, J., Palliser, H., Yates, D., Yawno, T., & Walker, D. (2008). Neurosteroids in the fetus and neonate: Potential protective role in compromised pregnancies. *Neurochem Int, 52*(4-5), 602-10. doi: 10.1016/j.neuint.2007.07.018

Ho, M., Bhatia, N., & Bhasin, S. (2004). Anabolic effects of androgens on muscles of female pelvic floor and lower urinary tract. *Curr Opin Obstet Gynecol, 16*(5), 405-9. doi: 10.1097/00001703-200410000-00009

Ho, S., Tang, W., Belmonte de Frausto, J., & Prins, G. (2006). Developmental exposure to estradiol and bisphenol A increases susceptibility to prostate carcinogenesis and epigenetically regulates phosphodiesterase type 4 variant 4. *Cancer Res, 66*(11), 5624-32. doi: 10.1158/0008-5472.CAN-06-0516

Hoberman, J., & Yesalis, C. (1995). The history of synthetic testosterone. *Sci Am, 272*(2), 76-81. doi:

10.1038/scientificamerican0295-76

Hoffman, M, DeWolf, W., & Morgentaler, A. (2000). Is low serum free testosterone a marker for high grade prostate cancer? *J Urol, 163*(3), 824-7.

Hogan, A., Kennelly, R., Collins, D., Baird, A., & Winter, D. (2009). Oestrogen inhibits human colonic motility by a non-genomic cell membrane receptor-dependent mechanism. *Br J Surg, 96*(7), 817-22. doi: 10.1002/bjs.6612

Holtorf, K. (2009). The bioidentical hormone debate: Are bioidentical hormones (estradiol, estriol, and progesterone) safer or more efficacious than commonly used synthetic versions in hormone replacement therapy? *Postgrad Med, 121*(1), 73-85. doi: 10.3810/pgm.2009.01.1949

Holzer, G., Riegler, E., Hönigsmann, H., Farokhnia, S., & Schmidt, J. (2005). Effects and side-effects of 2% progesterone cream on the skin of peri- and postmenopausal women: Results from a double-blind, vehicle-controlled, randomized study. *Br J Dermatol, 153*(3), 626-34. doi: 10.1111/j.1365-2133.2005.06685.x

Houck, J. (2003). "What do these women want?": Feminist responses to Feminine Forever, 1963-1980. *Bull Hist Med, 77*(1), 103-32. doi: 10.1353/bhm.2003.0023

Howard, J. (2007). Common factor of cancer and the metabolic syndrome may be low DHEA. *Ann Epidemiol, 17*(4), 270. doi: 10.1016/j.annepidem.2006.03.002

Hryb, D., Khan, M., Romas, N., & Rosner, W. (1995). The effect of extracts of the roots of the stinging nettle (Urtica dioica) on the interaction of SHBG with its receptor on human prostatic membranes. *Planta Med, 61*(1), 31-2. doi: 10.1055/s-2006-957993

Huang, A., Subak, L., Wing, R., West, D., Hernandez, A., Macer, J., & Grady, D. (2010). Program to reduce incontinence by diet and exercise investigators. An intensive behavioral weight loss intervention and hot flushes in women. *Arch Intern Med, 170*(13), 1161-7. doi: 10.1001/archinternmed.2010.162

Huang, V., Munarriz, R., & Goldstein, I. (2005). Bicycle riding and erectile dysfunction: An increase in interest (and concern). *J Sex Med, 2*(5), 596-604. doi: 10.1111/j.1743-6109.2005.00099.x

Huie, M. (1994). An acute myocardial infarction occurring in an anabolic steroid user. *Med Sci Sports Exerc, 26*(4), 408-13.

Hulley, S., Grady, D., Bush, T., Furberg, C., Herrington, D., Riggs, B., & Vittinghoff, E. (1998). Randomized trial of estrogen plus progestin for secondary prevention of coronary heart disease in postmenopausal women. Heart and Estrogen/progestin Replacement Study (HERS) Research Group. *JAMA, 280*(7), 605-13. doi: 10.1001/jama.280.7.605

Hunt, P., Gurnell, E., Huppert, F., Richards, C., Prevost, A., Wass, J., ... Chatterjee, V. (2000). Improvement in mood and fatigue after dehydroepiandrosterone replacement in Addison's disease in a randomized, double-blind trial. *J Clin Endocrinol Metab, 85*(12), 4650-6. doi: 10.1210/jcem.85.12.7022

Hurel, S., Koppiker, N., Newkirk, J., Close, P., Miller, M., Mardell, R., ... Kendall-Taylor, P. (1999). Relationship of physical exercise and ageing to growth hormone production. *Clin Endocrinol (Oxf), 51*(6), 687-91. doi: 10.1046/j.1365-2265.1999.00852.x

Hurley, B., Seals, D., Hagberg, J., Goldberg, A., Ostrove, S., Holloszy, J., ... Goldberg, A. (1984). High-density-lipoprotein cholesterol in bodybuilders v powerlifters. Negative effects of androgen use. *JAMA, 252*(4), 507-13.

Imhof, M., Gocan, A., Imhof, M., & Schmidt, M. (2018). Soy germ extract alleviates menopausal hot flushes: Placebo-controlled double-blind trial. *Eur J Clin Nutr, 72*(7), 961-970. doi: 10.1038/s41430-018-0173-3

Inotsuka, R., Uchimura, K., Yamatsu, A., Kim, M., & Katakura, Y. (2020). γ-Aminobutyric acid (GABA) activates neuronal cells by inducing the secretion of exosomes from intestinal cells. *Food Funct, 11*(10), 9285-9290. doi: 10.1039/d0fo01184c

Jankowska, E., Biel, B., Majda, J., Szklarska, A., Lopuszanska, M., Medras, M., ... Ponikowski, P. (2006). Anabolic deficiency in men with chronic heart failure: Prevalence and detrimental impact on survival. *Circulation, 114*(17), 1829-37. doi: 10.1161/CIRCULATIONAHA.106.649426

Jefferson, A. (2005). Phytoestrogens and the menopause – do they really help? *Nutrition Bulletin, 30*, 370-73. doi 10.1111/j.1467-3010.2005.00506.x

Jiang, Y., Miyazaki, T., Honda, A., Hirayama, T., Yoshida, S., Tanaka, N., & Matsuzaki, Y. (2005). Apoptosis and inhibition of the phosphatidylinositol 3-kinase/Akt signaling pathway in the anti-proliferative actions of dehydroepiandrosterone. *J Gastroenterol, 40*(5), 490-7. doi: 10.1007/s00535-005-1574-3

Kabat, G., Chang, C., Sparano, J., Sepkovie, D., Hu, X., Khalil, A., ... Bradlow, H. (1997). Urinary estrogen metabolites and breast cancer: a case-control study. *Cancer Epidemiol Biomarkers Prev, 6*(7), 505-9.

Kagan, L., & Dusek, J. (2006). Mind/body

interventions for hot flashes. *Menopause, 13*(5), 727-9. doi: 10.1097/01.gme.0000235365.57652.a3

Kaore, S., Langade, D., Yadav, V., Sharma, P., Thawani, V., & Sharma, R. (2012). Novel actions of progesterone: What we know today and what will be the scenario in the future? *J Pharm Pharmacol, 64*(8), 1040-62. doi: 10.1111/j.2042-7158.2012.01464.x

Kapoor, D., Goodwin, E., Channer, K., & Jones, T. (2006). Testosterone replacement therapy improves insulin resistance, glycaemic control, visceral adiposity and hypercholesterolaemia in hypogonadal men with type 2 diabetes. *Eur J Endocrinol, 154*(6), 899-906. doi: 10.1530/eje.1.02166

Kapoor, D., Malkin, C., Channer, K., & Jones, T. (2005). Androgens, insulin resistance and vascular disease in men. *Clin Endocrinol (Oxf), 63*(3), 239-50. doi: 10.1111/j.1365-2265.2005.02299.x

Karalis, K., Goodwin, G., & Majzoub, J. (1996). Cortisol blockade of progesterone: A possible molecular mechanism involved in the initiation of human labor. *Nat Med, 2*(5), 556-60. doi: 10.1038/nm0596-556

Kargozar, R., Azizi, H., & Salari, R. (2017). A review of effective herbal medicines in controlling menopausal symptoms. *Electron Physician, 9*(11), 5826-5833. doi:

10.19082/5826

Katalinic, A., & Rawal, R. (2008). Decline in breast cancer incidence after decrease in utilisation of hormone replacement therapy. *Breast Cancer Res Treat, 107*(3), 427-30. doi: 10.1007/s10549-007-9566-z

Kaur, P., Jodhka, P., Underwood, W., Bowles, C., de Fiebre, N., de Fiebre, C., & Singh, M. (2007). Progesterone increases brain-derived neuroptrophic factor expression and protects against glutamate toxicity in a mitogen-activated protein kinase- and phosphoinositide-3 kinase-dependent manner in cerebral cortical explants. *J Neurosci Res, 85*(11), 2441-9. doi: 10.1002/jnr.21370

Kawano, H., Yasue, H., Kitagawa, A., Hirai, N., Yoshida, T., Soejima, H., … Ogawa, H. (2003). Dehydroepiandrosterone supplementation improves endothelial function and insulin sensitivity in men. *J Clin Endocrinol Metab, 88*(7), 3190-5. doi: 10.1210/jc.2002-021603

Kelly, G. (2000). Peripheral metabolism of thyroid hormones: A review. *Altern Med Rev, 5*(4), 306-33.

Kenfield, S., DuPre, N., Richman, E., Stampfer, M., Chan, J., & Giovannucci, E. (2014). Mediterranean diet and prostate cancer risk and mortality in the Health Professionals Follow-up Study. *Eur Urol, 65*(5), 887-

94. doi: 10.1016/j.eururo.2013.08.009

Khan, T., Wu, D., & Dolzhenko, A. (2018). Effectiveness of fenugreek as a galactagogue: A network meta-analysis. *Phytother Res, 32*(3), 402-412. doi: 10.1002/ptr.5972

Khera, M., & Lipshultz, L. (2007). The role of testosterone replacement therapy following radical prostatectomy. *Urol Clin North Am, 34*(4), 549-53, vi. doi: 10.1016/j.ucl.2007.08.007

Kim, J., Jang, J., & Lee, S. (2021). An updated comprehensive review on vitamin A and carotenoids in breast cancer: Mechanisms, genetics, assessment, current evidence, and future clinical implications. *Nutrients, 13*(9). 3162. doi: 10.3390/nu13093162

Kim, J., Noh, W., Kim, A., Choi, Y., & Kim, Y. (2023). The effect of fenugreek in type 2 diabetes and prediabetes: A systematic review and meta-analysis of randomized controlled trials. *Int J Mol Sci, 24*(18), 13999. doi: 10.3390/ijms241813999

Klip, H., Verloop, J., van Gool, J., Koster, M., Burger, C., & van Leeuwen, F.(2002). OMEGA Project Group. Hypospadias in sons of women exposed to diethylstilbestrol in utero: A cohort study. *Lancet, 359*(9312), 1102-7. doi: 10.1016/S0140-6736(02)08152-7

Klotz, T., Mathers, M., Braun, M., Bloch, W., & Engelmann, U. (1999). Effectiveness of oral L-arginine in first-line treatment of erectile dysfunction in a controlled crossover study. *Urol Int, 63*(4), 220-3. doi: 10.1159/000030454

Koefoed, P., & Brahm, J. (1994). The permeability of the human red cell membrane to steroid sex hormones. *Biochim Biophys Acta, 1195*(1), 55-62. doi: 10.1016/0005-2736(94)90009-4

Koo, S., Ahn, Y., Lim, J., Cho, J., & Park, H. (2017). Obesity associates with vasomotor symptoms in postmenopause but with physical symptoms in perimenopause: A cross-sectional study. *BMC Womens Health, 17*(1), 126. doi: 10.1186/s12905-017-0487-7

Kraemer, W., Häkkinen, K., Newton, R., Nindl, B., Volek, J., McCormick, M., ... Evans, W. (1999). Effects of heavy-resistance training on hormonal response patterns in younger vs. older men. *J Appl Physiol (1985), 87*(3), 982-92. doi: 10.1152/jappl.1999.87.3.982

Kucuk, O., Sarkar, F., Djuric, Z., Sakr, W., Pollak, M., Khachik, F., ... Wood, D. Jr. (2002). Effects of lycopene supplementation in patients with localized prostate cancer. *Exp Biol Med (Maywood), 227*(10), 881-5. doi: 10.1177/153537020222701007

Kunelius, P., Lukkarinen, O., Hannuksela, M., Itkonen, O., & Tapanainen, J. (2002). The effects of transdermal dihydrotestosterone in the aging male: A prospective, randomized, double blind study. *J Clin Endocrinol Metab, 87*(4), 1467-72. doi: 10.1210/jcem.87.4.8138

La Vecchia, C., Franceschi, S., Parazzini, F., Regallo, M., Decarli, A., Gallus, G., …Tognoni, G. (1985). Benign breast disease and consumption of beverages containing methylxanthines. *J Natl Cancer Inst, 74*(5), 995-1000.

Lasco, A., Frisina, N., Morabito, N., Gaudio, A., Morini, E., Trifiletti, A., … Cucinotta, D. (2001). Metabolic effects of dehydroepiandrosterone replacement therapy in postmenopausal women. *Eur J Endocrinol, 145*(4), 457-61. doi: 10.1530/eje.0.1450457

Laudat, M., Cerdas, S., Fournier, C., Guiban, D., Guilhaume, B., & Luton, J. (1988). Salivary cortisol measurement: A practical approach to assess pituitary-adrenal function. *J Clin Endocrinol Metab, 66*(2), 343-8. doi: 10.1210/jcem-66-2-343

Laughlin, G., Barrett-Connor, E., Kritz-Silverstein, D., & von Mühlen, D. (2000). Hysterectomy, oophorectomy, and endogenous sex hormone levels in older women: The Rancho Bernardo Study. *J Clin*

Endocrinol Metab, 85(2), 645-51. doi: 10.1210/jcem.85.2.6405

Leake, A., Chisholm, G., & Habib, F. (1984). The effect of zinc on the 5 alpha-reduction of testosterone by the hyperplastic human prostate gland. *J Steroid Biochem, 20*(2), 651-5. doi: 10.1016/0022-4731(84)90138-9

Lebbink, J., Fish, A., Reumer, A., Natrajan, G., Winterwerp, H., & Sixma, T. (2010). Magnesium coordination controls the molecular switch function of DNA mismatch repair protein MutS. *J Biol Chem, 285*(17), 13131-41. doi: 10.1074/jbc.M109.066001

Lebret, T., Hervé, J., Gorny, P., Worcel, M., & Botto, H. (2002). Efficacy and safety of a novel combination of L-arginine glutamate and yohimbine hydrochloride: A new oral therapy for erectile dysfunction. *Eur Urol, 41*(6), 608-13; discussion 613. doi: 10.1016/s0302-2838(02)00175-6

Lee, J. (1991). Is natural progesterone the missing link in osteoporosis prevention and treatment? *Med Hypotheses, 35*(4), 316-8. doi: 10.1016/0306-9877(91)90276-5

Lee. J. R., & Hopkins, V. (2004). *What your doctor may not tell you about menopause: The breakthrough book on hormone balance* (2nd ed.). Warner Books: New York, NY.

Leisegang, K., Finelli, R., Sikka, S., & Panner Selvam, M. (2022). *Eurycoma longifolia* (Jack) improves serum total testosterone in men: A systematic review and meta-analysis of clinical trials. *Medicina (Kaunas), 58*(8), 1047. doi: 10.3390/medicina58081047

Leitão, A., Vieira, M., Pelegrini, A., da Silva, E., & Guimarães, A. (2021). A 6-month, double-blind, placebo-controlled, randomized trial to evaluate the effect of Eurycoma longifolia (Tongkat Ali) and concurrent training on erectile function and testosterone levels in androgen deficiency of aging males (ADAM). *Maturitas, 145*, 78-85. doi: 10.1016/j.maturitas.2020.12.002

Leo, J., Guo, C., Woon, C., Aw, S., & Lin, V. (2004). Glucocorticoid and mineralocorticoid cross-talk with progesterone receptor to induce focal adhesion and growth inhibition in breast cancer cells. *Endocrinology, 145*(3), 1314-21. doi: 10.1210/en.2003-0732

Leonard, L., Choi, M., & Cross, T. (2022). Maximizing the estrogenic potential of soy isoflavones through the gut microbiome: Implication for cardiometabolic health in postmenopausal women. *Nutrients, 14*(3), 553. doi: 10.3390/nu14030553

Leonetti, H., Landes, J., Steinberg, D., & Anasti, J. (2005). Transdermal progesterone cream as an alternative progestin in hormone therapy. *Altern Ther Health Med, 11*(6), 36-8

Lewis, S., Heaton, K., Oakey, R., & McGarrigle, H. (1997). Lower serum oestrogen concentrations associated with faster intestinal transit. *Br J Cancer, 76*(3), 395-400. doi: 10.1038/bjc.1997.397

Lewis, S., Oakey, R., & Heaton, K. (1998). Intestinal absorption of oestrogen: The effect of altering transit-time. *Eur J Gastroenterol Hepatol, 10*(1), 33-9. doi: 10.1097/00042737-199801000-00007

L'hermite, M., Simoncini, T., Fuller, S., & Genazzani, A. (2008). Could transdermal estradiol + progesterone be a safer postmenopausal HRT? A review. *Maturitas, 60*(3-4), 185-201. doi: 10.1016/j.maturitas.2008.07.007

Liske, E. (1998). Therapeutic efficacy and safety of Cimicifuga racemosa for gynecologic disorders. *Adv Ther, 15*(1), 45-53

Liu, D., & Dillon, J. (2002). Dehydroepiandrosterone activates endothelial cell nitric-oxide synthase by a specific plasma membrane receptor coupled to Galpha (i2,3). *J Biol Chem, 277*(24), 21379-88. doi: 10.1074/jbc.M200491200

Liu, Y. (2013). [Cardiovascular-protective effect of tadalafil in the treatment of erectile dysfunction].

Zhonghua Nan Ke Xue, 19(12), 1147-51. Chinese.

Lobo, R., Rosen, R., Yang, H., Block, B., & Van Der Hoop, R. (2003). Comparative effects of oral esterified estrogens with and without methyltestosterone on endocrine profiles and dimensions of sexual function in postmenopausal women with hypoactive sexual desire. *Fertil Steril, 79*(6), 1341-52. doi: 10.1016/s0015-0282(03)00358-3

Lock, M. (1998). Menopause: Lessons from anthropology. *Psychosom Med, 60*(4), 410-9. doi: 10.1097/00006842-199807000-00005

Longcope, C., Feldman, H., McKinlay, J., & Araujo, A. (2000). Diet and sex hormone-binding globulin. *J Clin Endocrinol Metab, 85*(1), 293-6. doi: 10.1210/jcem.85.1.6291

Lopatkin, N., Sivkov, A., Walther, C., Schläfke, S., Medvedev, A., Avdeichuk, J., … Engelmann, U. (2005). Long-term efficacy and safety of a combination of sabal and urtica extract for lower urinary tract symptoms--a placebo-controlled, double-blind, multicenter trial. *World J Urol, 23*(2), 139-46. doi: 10.1007/s00345-005-0501-9

Low, W.. & Tan, H. (2007). Asian traditional medicine for erectile dysfunction. *Journal of Men's Health & Gender, 4*(3), 245-250. Doi:

10.1016/j.jmhg.2007.o5.010

Lu, P, Masterman, D., Mulnard, R., Cotman, C., Miller, B., Yaffe, K., ... Cummings, J. (2006). Effects of testosterone on cognition and mood in male patients with mild Alzheimer disease and healthy elderly men. *Arch Neurol, 63*(2), 177-85. doi: 10.1001/archneur.63.2.nct50002

Ly, L., Jimenez, M., Zhuang, T., Celermajer, D., Conway, A., & Handelsman, D. (2001). A double-blind, placebo-controlled, randomized clinical trial of transdermal dihydrotestosterone gel on muscular strength, mobility, and quality of life in older men with partial androgen deficiency. *J Clin Endocrinol Metab, 86*(9), 4078-88. doi: 10.1210/jcem.86.9.7821

Lydeking-Olsen, E., Beck-Jensen, J., Setchell, K., & Holm-Jensen, T. (2004). Soymilk or progesterone for prevention of bone loss--a 2 year randomized, placebo-controlled trial. *Eur J Nutr, 43*(4), 246-57. doi: 10.1007/s00394-004-0497-8

MacLennan, A., MacLennan, A., & Wilson, D. (1993). The prevalence of hysterectomy in South Australia. *Med J Aust, 158*(12), 807-9. doi: 10.5694/j.1326-5377.1993.tb137666.x

MacNamara, P., O'Shaughnessy, C., Manduca, P., & Loughrey, H. (1995). Progesterone receptors are expressed in human osteoblast-like cell lines and in primary human osteoblast cultures. *Calcif Tissue Int, 57*(6), 436-41. doi: 10.1007/BF00301947

Madeiro, A., Girão, M., Sartori, M., Acquaroli, R., Baracat, E., & Rodrigues De Lima, G. (2002). Effects of the association of androgen/estrogen on the bladder and urethra of castrated rats. *Clin Exp Obstet Gynecol, 29*(2), 117-20

Malkin, C., Pugh, P., Jones, R., Jones, T., & Channer, K. (2003). Testosterone as a protective factor against atherosclerosis--immunomodulation and influence upon plaque development and stability. *J Endocrinol, 178*(3), 373-80. doi: 10.1677/joe.0.1780373

Malkin, C., Pugh, P., Jones, R., Kapoor, D., Channer, K., & Jones, T. (2004). The effect of testosterone replacement on endogenous inflammatory cytokines and lipid profiles in hypogonadal men. *J Clin Endocrinol Metab, 89*(7), 3313-8. doi: 10.1210/jc.2003-031069

Manson, J., Hsia, J., Johnson, K., Rossouw, J., Assaf, A., Lasser, N., ... Cushman, M. (2003). Women's Health Initiative Investigators. Estrogen plus progestin and the risk of coronary heart disease. *N Engl J Med, 349*(6), 523-34. doi: 10.1056/NEJMoa030808

Mansoori, A., Hosseini, S., Zilaee, M., Hormoznejad, R.,

& Fathi, M. (2020). Effect of fenugreek extract supplement on testosterone levels in male: A meta-analysis of clinical trials. *Phytother Res, 34*(7), 1550-1555. doi: 10.1002/ptr.6627

Marks, L., Mazer, N., Mostaghel, E., Hess, D., Dorey, F., Epstein, J., ... Nelson, P. (2006). Effect of testosterone replacement therapy on prostate tissue in men with late-onset hypogonadism: A randomized controlled trial. *JAMA, 296*(19),2351-61. doi: 10.1001/jama.296.19.2351

Martin, M., Block, J., Sanchez, S., Arnaud, C., & Beyene, Y. (1993). Menopause without symptoms: The endocrinology of menopause among rural Mayan Indians. *Am J Obstet Gynecol, 168*(6 Pt 1), 1839-43; discussion 1843-5. doi: 10.1016/0002-9378(93)90699-j

Martínez-Jabaloyas, J., Queipo-Zaragozá, A., Pastor-Hernández, F., Gil-Salom, M., & Chuan-Nuez, P. (2006). Testosterone levels in men with erectile dysfunction. *BJU Int, 97*(6), 1278-83. doi: 10.1111/j.1464-410X.2006.06154.x

Maruti, S., Lampe, J., Potter, J., Ready, A., & White, E. (2008). A prospective study of bowel motility and related factors on breast cancer risk. *Cancer Epidemiol Biomarkers Prev, 17*(7), 1746-50. doi: 10.1158/1055-9965.EPI-07-2850

Mattos, G., Heinzmann, J., Norkowski, S., Helbling, J., Minni, A., Moisan, M., & Touma, C. (2013). Corticosteroid-binding globulin contributes to the neuroendocrine phenotype of mice selected for extremes in stress reactivity. *J Endocrinol, 219*(3), 217-29. doi: 10.1530/JOE-13-0255

Maydych, V., Claus, M., Watzl, C., & Kleinsorge, T. (2018). Attention to emotional information is associated with cytokine responses to psychological stress. *Front Neurosci, 12*, 687. doi: 10.3389/fnins.2018.00687

Mayo, W., Le Moal, M., & Abrous, D. (2001). Pregnenolone sulfate and aging of cognitive functions: behavioral, neurochemical, and morphological investigations. *Horm Behav, 40*(2), 215-7. doi: 10.1006/hbeh.2001.1677

McCallum, K., & Reading, C. (1989). Hot flushes are induced by thermogenic stimuli. *Br J Urol, 64*(5), 507-10. doi: 10.1111/j.1464-410x.1989.tb05288.x

McCormack, P., Reed, H., Thomas, J., & Malik, M. (1996). Increase in rT3 serum levels observed during extended Alaskan field operations of Naval personnel. *Alaska Med, 38*(3), 89-97.

McKenzie, R., O'Fallon, A., Dale, J., Demitrack, M., Sharma, G., Deloria, M., … Straus, S. (1998). Low-
523

dose hydrocortisone for treatment of chronic fatigue syndrome: A randomized controlled trial. *JAMA, 280*(12), 1061-6. doi: 10.1001/jama.280.12.1061

McTernan, P., Anderson, L., Anwar, A., Eggo, M., Crocker, J., Barnett, A., ... Kumar, S. (2002). Glucocorticoid regulation of p450 aromatase activity in human adipose tissue: Gender and site differences. *J Clin Endocrinol Metab, 87*(3), 1327-36. doi: 10.1210/jcem.87.3.8288

McTernan, P., Anwar, A., Eggo, M., Barnett, A., Stewart, P., & Kumar, S. (2000). Gender differences in the regulation of P450 aromatase expression and activity in human adipose tissue. *Int J Obes Relat Metab Disord, 24*(7), 875-81. doi: 10.1038/sj.ijo.0801254

Meier, C., Nguyen, T., Handelsman, D., Schindler, C., Kushnir, M., Rockwood, A., ... Seibel, M. (2008). Endogenous sex hormones and incident fracture risk in older men: The Dubbo Osteoporosis Epidemiology Study. *Arch Intern Med, 168*(1), 47-54. doi: 10.1001/archinternmed.2007.2

Meissner, H., Reich-Bilinska, H., Mscisz, A., & Kedzia, B. (2006). Therapeutic effects of pre-gelatinized maca (Lepidium Peruvianum Chacon) used as a non-hormonal alternative to HRT in perimenopausal women

- clinical pilot study. *Int J Biomed Sci, 2*(2), 143-59.

Meldrum, D., Davidson, B., Tataryn, I., & Judd, H. (1981). Changes in circulating steroids with aging in postmenopausal women. *Obstet Gynecol, 57*(5), 624-8.

Merkulov, V., Merkulova, T., & Bondar, N. (2017). Mechanisms of brain glucocorticoid resistance in stress-induced psychopathologies. *Biochemistry (Mosc), 82*(3), 351-365. doi: 10.1134/S0006297917030142

Mewis, C., Spyridopoulos, I., Kühlkamp, V., & Seipel, L. (1996). Manifestation of severe coronary heart disease after anabolic drug abuse. *Clin Cardiol, 19*(2), 153-5. doi: 10.1002/clc.4960190216

Michnovicz, J., Adlercreutz, H., & Bradlow, H. (1997). Changes in levels of urinary estrogen metabolites after oral indole-3-carbinol treatment in humans. *J Natl Cancer Inst, 89*(10), 718-23. doi: 10.1093/jnci/89.10.718

Minton, J., Abou-Issa, H., Reiches, N., & Roseman, J. (1981). Clinical and biochemical studies on methylxanthine-related fibrocystic breast disease. *Surgery, 90*(2), 299-304.

Mirzaee, F., Fakari, F., Babakhanian, M., Roozbeh, N., & Ghazanfarpour, M. (2022). The effectiveness of herbal medicines on cyclic mastalgia: A systematic review on meta-analysis. *Rev Bras Ginecol Obstet,* *44*(10), 972-985. doi: 10.1055/s-0042-1755456

Miyagawa, K., Rösch, J., Stanczyk, F., & Hermsmeyer, K. (1997). Medroxyprogesterone interferes with ovarian steroid protection against coronary vasospasm. *Nat Med,* (3), 324-7. doi: 10.1038/nm0397-324

Mohr, P., Wang, D., Gregory, W., Richards, M., & Fentiman, I. (1996). Serum progesterone and prognosis in operable breast cancer. *Br J Cancer,* *73*(12), 1552-5. doi: 10.1038/bjc.1996.292

Moncrieff, J., Cooper, R., Stockmann, T., Amendola, S., Hengartner, M., & Horowitz, M. (2023). The serotonin theory of depression: a systematic umbrella review of the evidence. *Mol Psychiatry,* *28*(8), 3243-3256. doi: 10.1038/s41380-022-01661-0

Money, S., Muss, W., Thelmo, W., Boeckl, O., Pimpl, W., Kaindl, H., ... Jaffe B., et al. (1989). Immunocytochemical localization of estrogen and progesterone receptors in human thyroid. *Surgery,* *106*(6), 975-8; discussion 979.

Mónica, F., & De Nucci, G. (2019). Tadalafil for the treatment of benign prostatic hyperplasia. *Expert Opin Pharmacother,* *20*(8), 929-937. doi: 10.1080/14656566.2019.1589452

Monteleone, P., Beinat, L., Tanzillo, C., Maj, M., & Kemali, D. (1990). Effects of phosphatidylserine on the neuroendocrine response to physical stress in humans. *Neuroendocrinology, 52*(3), 243-8. doi: 10.1159/000125593

Monteleone, P., Maj, M., Beinat, L., Natale, M., & Kemali, D. (1992). Blunting by chronic phosphatidylserine administration of the stress-induced activation of the hypothalamo-pituitary-adrenal axis in healthy men. *Eur J Clin Pharmacol, 42*(4), 385-8. doi: 10.1007/BF00280123

Morales, A., Nolan, J., Nelson, J., & Yen, S. (1994). Effects of replacement dose of dehydroepiandrosterone in men and women of advancing age. *J Clin Endocrinol Metab, 78*(6), 1360-7. doi: 10.1210/jcem.78.6.7515387

Morgan, C. 3rd, Southwick, S., Hazlett, G., Rasmusson, A., Hoyt, G., Zimolo, Z., & Charney, D. (2004). Relationships among plasma dehydroepiandrosterone sulfate and cortisol levels, symptoms of dissociation, and objective performance in humans exposed to acute stress. *Arch Gen Psychiatry, 61*(8), 819-25. doi: 10.1001/archpsyc.61.8.819

Morgentaler, A. (2007). Testosterone replacement therapy and prostate cancer. *Urol Clin North Am, 34*(4), 555-63, vii. doi: 10.1016/j.ucl.2007.08.002

Morgentaler, A. Abello, A., & Bubley, G. (2021). Testosterone therapy in men with biochemical recurrence and metastatic prostate cancer: Initial observations. *Andro Clin Res Ther, 2*:1, 121-128. doi: 10.1089/andro.2021.000

Moskowitz, D. (2006). A comprehensive review of the safety and efficacy of bioidentical hormones for the management of menopause and related health risks. *Altern Med Rev, 11*(3), 208-23.

Moynihan, R., & Cassels, A. (2005). Selling Sickness How the Drug Companies are turning us all into patients. Publ Allen & Unwin. ISBN 1 74114 579 1

Mulnard, R., Cotman, C., Kawas, C., van Dyck, C., Sano, M., Doody, R., … Thal, L. (2000). Estrogen replacement therapy for treatment of mild to moderate Alzheimer disease: A randomized controlled trial. Alzheimer's Disease Cooperative Study. *JAMA, 283*(8), 1007-15. doi: 10.1001/jama.283.8.1007

Myers, G. (1951). Pregnenolone in the treatment of rheumatoid arthritis. *Ann Rheum Dis, 10*(1), 32-45. doi: 10.1136/ard.10.1.32

Nagulapalli Venkata, K., Swaroop, A., Bagchi, D., & Bishayee, A. (2017). A small plant with big benefits: Fenugreek (Trigonella foenum-graecum Linn.) for disease prevention and health promotion. *Mol Nutr Food*

Res, 61(6), doi: 10.1002/mnfr.201600950

Nair, K., Rizza, R., O'Brien, P., Dhatariya, K., Short, K., Nehra, A., ... Jensen, M. (2006). DHEA in elderly women and DHEA or testosterone in elderly men. *N Engl J Med, 355*(16), 1647-59. doi: 10.1056/NEJMoa054629

Nakhla, A., Romas, N., & Rosner, W. (1997). Estradiol activates the prostate androgen receptor and prostate-specific antigen secretion through the intermediacy of sex hormone-binding globulin. *J Biol Chem, 272*(11), 6838-41. doi: 10.1074/jbc.272.11.6838

Nelson, D., Sammel, M., Freeman, E., Lin, H., Gracia, C., & Schmitz, K. (2008). Effect of physical activity on menopausal symptoms among urban women. *Med Sci Sports Exerc, 40*(1), 50-8. doi: 10.1249/mss.0b013e318159d1e4

Nelson, R. (2002). Steroidal oestrogens added to list of known human carcinogens. *Lancet, 360*(9350), 2053. doi: 10.1016/S0140-6736(02)12045-9

Nettleship, J., Jones, R., Channer, K., & Jones, T. (2009). Testosterone and coronary artery disease. *Front Horm Res, 37*, 91-107. doi: 10.1159/000176047

Neychev, V., & Mitev, V. (2005). The aphrodisiac herb Tribulus terrestris does not influence the androgen production in young men. *J Ethnopharmacol, 101*(1-3), 319-23. doi: 10.1016/j.jep.2005.05.017

Nishiyama, T., Ikarashi, T., Hashimoto, Y., Suzuki, K., & Takahashi, K. (2006). Association between the dihydrotestosterone level in the prostate and prostate cancer aggressiveness using the Gleason score. *J Urol, 176*(4 Pt 1), 1387-91. doi: 10.1016/j.juro.2006.06.066

Ohta, Y., Mitani, F., Ishimura, Y., Yanagibashi, K., Kawamura, M., & Kawato, S. (1990). Conversion of cholesterol to pregnenolone mobilizes cytochrome P-450 in the inner membrane of adrenocortical mitochondria: Protein rotation study. *J Biochem, 107*(1), 97-104. doi: 10.1093/oxfordjournals.jbchem.a123020

Ojumu, A., & Dobs, A. (2003). Is hypogonadism a risk factor for sexual dysfunction? *J Androl, 24*(6 Suppl), S46-51. doi: 10.1002/j.1939-4640.2003.tb02746.x

Okamoto, R., & Leibfritz, D. (1997). Adverse effects of reverse triiodothyronine on cellular metabolism as assessed by 1H and 31P NMR spectroscopy. *Res Exp Med (Berl), 197*(4), 211-7. doi: 10.1007/s004330050070

Oktem, M., Eroglu, D., Karahan, H., Taskintuna, N., Kuscu, E., & Zeyneloglu, H. (2007). Black cohosh and fluoxetine in the treatment of postmenopausal symptoms: a prospective, randomized trial. *Adv Ther,* *24*(2), 448-61. doi: 10.1007/BF02849914

Oliveira, C., Moraes, M., Moraes, M., Bezerra, F., Abib, E., & De Nucci, G. (2005). Clinical toxicology study of an herbal medicinal extract of Paullinia cupana, Trichilia catigua, Ptychopetalum olacoides and Zingiber officinale (Catuama) in healthy volunteers. *Phytother Res, 19*(1), 54-7. doi: 10.1002/ptr.1484

Olsson, H., Ingvar, C., & Bladström, A. (2003). Hormone replacement therapy containing progestins and given continuously increases breast carcinoma risk in Sweden. *Cancer, 97*(6), 1387-92. doi: 10.1002/cncr.11205

Om, A., & Chung, K. (1996). Dietary zinc deficiency alters 5 alpha-reduction and aromatization of testosterone and androgen and estrogen receptors in rat liver. *J Nutr, 126*(4), 842-8. doi: 10.1093/jn/126.4.842

Osawa, E., Nakajima, A., Yoshida, S., Omura, M., Nagase, H., Ueno, N., ... Sekihara, H. (2002). Chemoprevention of precursors to colon cancer by dehydroepiandrosterone (DHEA). *Life Sci, 70*(22), 2623-30. doi: 10.1016/s0024-3205(02)01521-7

Osman, I., Drobnjak, M., Fazzari, M., Ferrara, J., Scher, H., & Cordon-Cardo, C. (1999). Inactivation of the p53 pathway in prostate cancer: impact on tumor progression. *Clin Cancer Res, 5*(8), 2082-8

Osmers, R., Friede, M., Liske, E., Schnitker, J., Freudenstein, J., & Henneicke-von Zepelin, H. (2005). Efficacy and safety of isopropanolic black cohosh extract for climacteric symptoms. *Obstet Gynecol, 105*(5 Pt 1), 1074-83. doi: 10.1097/01.AOG.0000158865.98070.89

Page, J., Colditz, G., Rifai, N., Barbieri, R., Willett, W., & Hankinson, S. (2004). Plasma adrenal androgens and risk of breast cancer in premenopausal women. *Cancer Epidemiol Biomarkers Prev, 13*(6), 1032-6.

Palmer, J., Wise., L., Hatch, E., Troisi, R., Titus-Ernstoff, L., Strohsnitter, W., ... Hoover, R. (2006) Prenatal diethylstilbestrol exposure and risk of breast cancer. *Cancer Epidemiol Biomarkers Prev, 15*(8), 1509-14. doi: 10.1158/1055-9965.EPI-06-0109

Papasozomenos, S., & Shanavas, A. (2002). Testosterone prevents the heat shock-induced overactivation of glycogen synthase kinase-3 beta but not of cyclin-dependent kinase 5 and c-Jun NH2-terminal kinase and concomitantly abolishes hyperphosphorylation of tau: implications for Alzheimer's disease. *Proc Natl Acad Sci U S A, 99*(3), 1140-5. doi: 10.1073/pnas.032646799

Phillips, T., Symons, J., & Menon, S. (2008). HT Study

Group. Does hormone therapy improve age-related skin changes in postmenopausal women? A randomized, double-blind, double-dummy, placebo-controlled multicenter study assessing the effects of norethindrone acetate and ethinyl estradiol in the improvement of mild to moderate age-related skin changes in postmenopausal women. *J Am Acad Dermatol, 59*(3), 397-404.e3. doi: 10.1016/j.jaad.2008.05.009

Pillsworth, E., Haselton, M., & Buss, D. (2004). Ovulatory shifts in female sexual desire. *J Sex Res, 41*(1), 55-65. doi: 10.1080/00224490409552213

Pitteloud, N., Hardin, M., Dwyer, A., Valassi, E., Yialamas, M., Elahi, D., & Hayes, F. (2005). Increasing insulin resistance is associated with a decrease in Leydig cell testosterone secretion in men. *J Clin Endocrinol Metab, 90*(5), 2636-41. doi: 10.1210/jc.2004-219

Pollard, M., Snyder, D., & Luckert, P. (1987). Dihydrotestosterone does not induce prostate adenocarcinoma in L-W rats. *Prostate, 10*(4), 325-31. doi: 10.1002/pros.2990100406

Pranjić, N., Nuhbegović, S., Brekalo-Lazarević, S., & Kurtić, A. (2012). Is adrenal exhaustion synonym of syndrome burnout at workplace? *Coll Antropol, 36*(3), 911-9.

Prehn, R. (1999). On the prevention and therapy of prostate cancer by androgen administration. *Cancer Res, 59*(17), 4161-4.

Price, J., & Leng, G. (2012). Steroid sex hormones for lower limb atherosclerosis. *Cochrane Database Syst Rev, 10*(10), CD000188. doi: 10.1002/14651858.CD000188. Update in: Cochrane Database Syst Rev. 2012;10:CD000188.

Prigent, H., Maxime, V., & Annane, D. (2003). Clinical review: Corticotherapy in sepsis. *Crit Care, 8*(2), 122-9. doi: 10.1186/cc2374

Prins, G., & Korach, K. (2008). The role of estrogens and estrogen receptors in normal prostate growth and disease. *Steroids, 73*(3), 233-44. doi: 10.1016/j.steroids.2007.10.013

Prior, J. (2018). Progesterone for the prevention and treatment of osteoporosis in women. *Climacteric, 21*(4), 366-374. doi: 10.1080/13697137.2018.1467400

Prior, J., Naess, M., Langhammer, A., & Forsmo, S. (2015). Ovulation Prevalence in Women with Spontaneous Normal-Length Menstrual Cycles - A Population-Based Cohort from HUNT3, Norway. *PLoS One, 10*(8), e0134473. doi: 10.1371/journal.pone.0134473

Prior, J., Vigna, Y., Barr, S., Rexworthy, C., & Lentle, B. (1994). Cyclic medroxyprogesterone treatment increases bone density: A controlled trial in active women with menstrual cycle disturbances. *Am J Med, 96*(6), 521-30. doi: 10.1016/0002-9343(94)90092-2

Prior, J., Vigna, Y., Schechter, M., & Burgess, A. (1990). Spinal bone loss and ovulatory disturbances. *N Engl J Med, 323*(18), 1221-7. doi: 10.1056/NEJM199011013231801

Prior, J., Vigna, Y., Wark, J., Eyre, D., Lentle, B., Li, D., … Atley, L. (1997). Premenopausal ovariectomy-related bone loss: A randomized, double-blind, one-year trial of conjugated estrogen or medroxyprogesterone acetate. *J Bone Miner Res, 12*(11), 1851-63. doi: 10.1359/jbmr.1997.12.11.1851

Prossnitz, E., Arterburn, J., Smith, H., Oprea, T., Sklar, L., & Hathaway, H. (2008). Estrogen signaling through the transmembrane G protein-coupled receptor GPR30. *Annu Rev Physiol, 70*, 165-90. doi: 10.1146/annurev.physiol.70.113006.100518

Putman, P., Hermans, E., Koppeschaar, H., van Schijndel, A., & van Honk, J. (2007). A single administration of cortisol acutely reduces preconscious attention for fear in anxious young men. *Psychoneuroendocrinology, 32*(7), 793-802. doi:

10.1016/j.psyneuen.2007.05.009

Qiu, D., Hu, J., Zhang, S., Cai, W., Miao, J., Li, P., & Jiang, W. (2024). Fenugreek extract improves diabetes-induced endothelial dysfunction *via* the arginase 1 pathway. *Food Funct, 15*(7), 3446-3462. doi: 10.1039/d3fo04283a

Raina, P., Santaguida, P., Ismaila, A., Patterson, C., Cowan, D., Levine, M., ... Oremus, M. (2008). Effectiveness of cholinesterase inhibitors and memantine for treating dementia: Evidence review for a clinical practice guideline. *Ann Intern Med, 148*(5), 379-97. doi: 10.7326/0003-4819-148-5-200803040-00009

Raisi, F., Farnia, V., Ghanbarian, N., & Ghafuri, Z. (2010). Effects of herbal vigRX on premature ejaculation: A randomized, double-blind study. *Iran J Psychiatry, 5*(1), 4-6.

Raison, C., & Miller, A. (2003). When not enough is too much: The role of insufficient glucocorticoid signaling in the pathophysiology of stress-related disorders. *Am J Psychiatry, 160*(9), 1554-65. doi: 10.1176/appi.ajp.160.9.1554

Rako, S. (1998). Testosterone deficiency: A key factor in the increased cardiovascular risk to women following hysterectomy or with natural aging? *J*

Womens Health, 7(7), 825-9. doi: 10.1089/jwh.1998.7.825

Rako, S. (2000). Testosterone supplemental therapy after hysterectomy with or without concomitant oophorectomy: Estrogen alone is not enough. *J Womens Health Gend Based Med, 9*(8), 917-23. doi: 10.1089/152460900750020955

Rao, A., Steels, E., Inder, W., Abraham, S., & Vitetta, L. (2016). Testofen, a specialised Trigonella foenum-graecum seed extract reduces age-related symptoms of androgen decrease, increases testosterone levels and improves sexual function in healthy aging males in a double-blind randomised clinical study. *Aging Male, 19*(2), 134-42. doi: 10.3109/13685538.2015.1135323

Rao, A., Steels, E., Beccaria, G., Inder, W., & Vitetta, L. (2015). Influence of a Specialized Trigonella foenum-graecum Seed Extract (Libifem), on Testosterone, Estradiol and Sexual Function in Healthy Menstruating Women, a Randomised Placebo Controlled Study. *Phytother Res, 29*(8), 1123-30. doi: 10.1002/ptr.5355

Ravdin, P., Cronin, K., Howlader, N., Berg, C., Chlebowski, R., Feuer, E., ... Berry, D. (2007). The decrease in breast-cancer incidence in 2003 in the United States. *N Engl J Med, 356*(16), 1670-4. doi: 10.1056/NEJMsr070105

Reed, G., Peterson, K., Smith, H., Gray, J., Sullivan, D., Mayo, M., … Hurwitz, A. (2005). A phase I study of indole-3-carbinol in women: Tolerability and effects. *Cancer Epidemiol Biomarkers Prev, 14*(8), 1953-60. doi: 10.1158/1055-9965.EPI-05-0121

Resnick, S., Espeland, M., Jaramillo, S., Hirsch, C., Stefanick, M., Murray, A., … Davatzikos, C. (2009). Postmenopausal hormone therapy and regional brain volumes: The WHIMS-MRI Study. *Neurology, 72*(2), 135-42. doi: 10.1212/01.wnl.0000339037.76336.cf

Rhoden, E., & Morgentaler, A. (2003) Testosterone replacement therapy in hypogonadal men at high risk for prostate cancer: Results of 1 year of treatment in men with prostatic intraepithelial neoplasia. *J Urol, 170*(6 Pt 1), 2348-51. doi: 10.1097/01.ju.0000091104.71869.8e

Riis, B., Thomsen, K., Strøm, V., & Christiansen, C. (1987). The effect of percutaneous estradiol and natural progesterone on postmenopausal bone loss. *Am J Obstet Gynecol, 156*(1), 61-5. doi: 10.1016/0002-9378(87)90203-1

Risbridger, G., Bianco, J., Ellem, S., & McPherson, S. (2003). Oestrogens and prostate cancer. *Endocr Relat Cancer, 10*(2), 187-91. doi: 10.1677/erc.0.0100187

Ritsner, M., Maayan, R., Gibel, A., & Weizman, A.

(2007). Differences in blood pregnenolone and dehydroepiandrosterone levels between schizophrenia patients and healthy subjects. *Eur Neuropsychopharmacol, 17*(5), 358-65. doi: 10.1016/j.euroneuro.2006.10.001

Rizk, D., Raaschou, T., Mason, N., & Berg, B. (2001). Evidence of progesterone receptors in the mucosa of the urinary bladder. *Scand J Urol Nephrol, 35*(4), 305-9. doi: 10.1080/003655901750425891

Rock, C., Flatt, S., Laughlin, G., Gold, E., Thomson, C., Natarajan, L., ... Pierce, J.(2008). Women's Healthy Eating and Living Study Group. Reproductive steroid hormones and recurrence-free survival in women with a history of breast cancer. *Cancer Epidemiol Biomarkers Prev, 17*(3), 614-20. doi: 10.1158/1055-9965.EPI-07-0761

Roddam, A., Allen, N., Appleby, P., & Key T. (2008). Endogenous Hormones and Prostate Cancer Collaborative Group. Endogenous sex hormones and prostate cancer: A collaborative analysis of 18 prospective studies. *J Natl Cancer Inst, 100*(3), 170-83. doi: 10.1093/jnci/djm323

Rogan, E. (2006). The natural chemopreventive compound indole-3-carbinol: State of the science. *In Vivo, 20*(2), 221-8.

Rogerson, S., Riches, C., Jennings, C., Weatherby, R., Meir, R., & Marshall-Gradisnik, S. (2007). The effect of five weeks of Tribulus terrestris supplementation on muscle strength and body composition during preseason training in elite rugby league players. *J Strength Cond Res, 21*(2), 348-53. doi: 10.1519/R-18395.1

Romani, W., Gallicchio, L., & Flaws, J. (2009). The association between physical activity and hot flash severity, frequency, and duration in mid-life women. *Am J Hum Biol, 21*(1):127-9. doi: 10., 002/ajhb.20834

Römmler, A. (2003). Adrenopause und dehydroepiandrosteron: pharmakotherapie versus substitution [Adrenopause and dehydroepiandrosterone: pharmacological therapy versus replacement therapy]. *Gynakol Geburtshilfliche Rundsch, 43*(2), 79-90. German. doi: 10.1159/000069165

Roney, J., & Simmons, Z. (2013). Hormonal predictors of sexual motivation in natural menstrual cycles. *Horm Behav, 63*(4), 636-45. doi: 10.1016/j.yhbeh.2013.02.013

Rossouw, J., Anderson, G., Prentice, R., LaCroix, A., Kooperberg, C., Stefanick, M., ... Ockene, J (2002). Writing Group for the Women's Health Initiative Investigators. Risks and benefits of estrogen plus progestin in healthy postmenopausal women: Principal results from the Women's Health Initiative randomized controlled trial. *JAMA, 288*(3), 321-33. doi: 10.1001/jama.288.3.321

Rothman, R., Leure-duPree, A., & Fosmire, G. (1986). Zinc deficiency affects the composition of the rat adrenal gland. *Proc Soc Exp Biol Med, 182*(3), 350-7. doi: 10.3181/00379727-182-42351

Rubello, D., Sonino, N., Casara, D., Girelli, M., Busnardo, B., & Boscaro, M. (1992). Acute and chronic effects of high glucocorticoid levels on hypothalamic-pituitary-thyroid axis in man. *J Endocrinol Invest, 15*(6), 437-41. doi: 10.1007/BF03348767

Sakamaki, K., Nomura, M., Yamato, K., & Tanaka, J. (2004). GABA-mediated attenuation of noradrenaline release in the rat median preoptic area caused by intravenous injection of metaraminol. *Auton Neurosci, 111*(1), 7-14. doi: 10.1016/j.autneu.2003.12.004

Saklayen, M. (2018). The global epidemic of the metabolic syndrome. *Curr Hypertens Rep, 20*(2), 12. doi: 10.1007/s11906-018-0812-z

Salke, R., Rowland, T., & Burke, E. (1985). Left ventricular size and function in body builders using anabolic steroids. *Med Sci Sports Exerc, 17*(6), 701-4. doi: 10.1249/00005768-198512000-00014

Samuels, M., & McDaniel, P. (1997). Thyrotropin levels during hydrocortisone infusions that mimic fasting-induced cortisol elevations: A clinical research center study. *J Clin Endocrinol Metab, 82*(11), 3700-4. doi: 10.1210/jcem.82.11.4376

Santamarina, R., Besocke, A., Romano, L., Ioli, P., & Gonorazky, S. (2008). Ischemic stroke related to anabolic abuse. *Clin Neuropharmacol, 31*(2), 80-5. doi: 10.1097/WNF.0b013e3180ed4485

Sapolsky, R. (2004). *Why zebras don't get ulcers* (3rd ed.). Holt Publishers: New York, NY.

Sator, P., Schmidt, J., Sator, M., Huber, J., & Hönigsmann, H. (2001). The influence of hormone replacement therapy on skin ageing: A pilot study. *Maturitas, 39*(1), 43-55. doi: 10.1016/s0378-5122(00)00225-5

Schelling, G., Roozendaal, B., & De Quervain, D. (2004). Can posttraumatic stress disorder be prevented with glucocorticoids? *Ann N Y Acad Sci, 1032*, 158-66. doi: 10.1196/annals.1314.013

Schmidt, P., Daly, R., Bloch, M., Smith, M., Danaceau, M., St Clair, L., … Rubinow, D. (2005). Dehydroepiandrosterone monotherapy in midlife-onset major and minor depression. *Arch Gen Psychiatry, 62*(2), 154-62. doi: 10.1001/archpsyc.62.2.154

Schumacher, M., Guennoun, R., Stein, D., & De Nicola, A. (2007). Progesterone: Therapeutic opportunities for neuroprotection and myelin repair. *Pharmacol Ther, 116*(1), 77-106. doi: 10.1016/j.pharmthera.2007.06.001

Schwab, R., Johnson, G., Housh, T., Kinder, J., & Weir, J. (1993). Acute effects of different intensities of weightlifting on serum testosterone. *Med Sci Sports Exerc, 25*(12), 1381-5.

Schwarz, S., Obermüller-Jevic, U., Hellmis, E., Koch, W., Jacobi, G., & Biesalski, H. (2008). Lycopene inhibits disease progression in patients with benign prostate hyperplasia. *J Nutr, 138*(1), 49-53. doi: 10.1093/jn/138.1.49

Selva, D., Hogeveen, K., Innis, S., & Hammond, G. (2007). Monosaccharide-induced lipogenesis regulates the human hepatic sex hormone-binding globulin gene. *J Clin Invest, 117*(12), 3979-87. doi: 10.1172/JCI32249

Sengupta, P., Agarwal, A., Pogrebetskaya, M., Roychoudhury, S., Durairajanayagam, D., & Henkel, R. (2018). Role of Withania somnifera (Ashwagandha) in the management of male infertility. *Reprod Biomed Online, 36*(3), 311-326. doi: 10.1016/j.rbmo.2017.11.007

Setlur, S., Mertz, K., Hoshida, Y., Demichelis, F.,

Lupien, M., Perner, S., ... Rubin, M. (2008). Estrogen-dependent signaling in a molecularly distinct subclass of aggressive prostate cancer. *J Natl Cancer Inst, 100*(11), 815-25. doi: 10.1093/jnci/djn150

Shabsigh, R. (2004). Testosterone therapy in erectile dysfunction. *Aging Male, 7*(4), 312-8. doi: 10.1080/13685530400016540

Shabsigh, R. (2005). Testosterone therapy in erectile dysfunction and hypogonadism. *J Sex Med, 2*(6), 785-92. doi: 10.1111/j.1743-6109.2005.00139.x

Shifren, J., Braunstein, G., Simon, J., Casson, P., Buster, J., Redmond, G., ... Mazer, N. (2000). Transdermal testosterone treatment in women with impaired sexual function after oophorectomy. *N Engl J Med, 343*(10), 682-8. doi: 10.1056/NEJM200009073431002

Shumaker, S., Legault, C., Kuller, L., Rapp, S., Thal, L., Lane, D., ... Coker, L.(2004). Women's Health Initiative Memory Study. Conjugated equine estrogens and incidence of probable dementia and mild cognitive impairment in postmenopausal women: Women's Health Initiative Memory Study. *JAMA, 291*(24), 2947-58. doi: 10.1001/jama.291.24.2947

Sievert, L., Freedman, R., Garcia, J., Foster, J., del Carmen Romano Soriano, M., Longcope, C., & Franz,

C. (2002). Measurement of hot flashes by sternal skin conductance and subjective hot flash report in Puebla, Mexico. *Menopause, 9*(5):3,7-76. doi: 10.1097/00042192-200209000-00010

Singh, M., & Su, C. (2013). Progesterone and neuroprotection. *Horm Behav, 63*(2), 284-90. doi: 10.1016/j.yhbeh.2012.06.003

Singh, N., Bhalla, M., de Jager, P., & Gilca, M. (2011). An overview on ashwagandha: a Rasayana (rejuvenator) of Ayurveda. *Afr J Tradit Complement Altern Med, 8*(5 Suppl), 208-13. doi: 10.4314/ajtcam.v8i5S.9

Singhal, H., Greene, M., Tarulli, G., Zarnke, A., Bourgo, R., Laine, M., ... Greene, G. (2016). Genomic agonism and phenotypic antagonism between estrogen and progesterone receptors in breast cancer. *Sci Adv, 2*(6), e1501924. doi: 10.1126/sciadv.1501924

Smith, D., Prentice, R., Thompson, D., & Herrmann, W. (1975). Association of exogenous estrogen and endometrial carcinoma. *N Engl J Med, 293*(23), 1164-7. doi: 10.1056/NEJM197512042932302

Snead, E. (1992). Some Call it AIDS ... I Call it Murder; Vol 1 and 2. AVM Publications, San Antonio, Texas.

Soares, N., Elias, M., Lima Machado, C., Trindade, B.,

Borojevic, R., & Teodoro, A. (2019). Comparative analysis of lycopene content from different tomato-based food products on the cellular activity of prostate cancer cell lines. *Foods, 8*(6), 201. doi: 10.3390/foods8060201

Sökeland, J. (2000). Combined sabal and urtica extract compared with finasteride in men with benign prostatic hyperplasia: Analysis of prostate volume and therapeutic outcome. *BJU Int, 86*(4), 439-42. doi: 10.1046/j.1464-410x.2000.00776.x

Soravia L., de Quervain, D., & Heinrichs, M. (2009). Glucocorticoids do not reduce subjective fear in healthy subjects exposed to social stress. *Biol Psychol, 81*(3), 184-8. doi: 10.1016/j.biopsycho.2009.04.001

Soravia, L., Heinrichs, M., Aerni, A., Maroni, C., Schelling, G., Ehlert, U., ... de Quervain, D. (2006). Glucocorticoids reduce phobic fear in humans. *Proc Natl Acad Sci U S A, 103*(14), 5585-90. doi: 10.1073/pnas.0509184103

Spark, M., Dunn, R., & Houlahan, K. (2009). Women's perspective on progesterone: A qualitative study conducted in Australia. *Int J Pharm Compd, 13*(4), 345-9.

Spark, R. (2007). Testosterone, diabetes mellitus, and the metabolic syndrome. *Curr Urol Rep, 8*(6), 467-71.

doi: 10.1007/s11934-007-0050-4

Srivatsav, A., Balasubramanian, A., Pathak, U., Rivera-Mirabal, J., Thirumavalavan, N., Hotaling, J., … Pastuszak, A. (2020). Efficacy and safety of common ingredients in aphrodisiacs used for erectile dysfunction: A review. *Sex Med Rev, 8*(3), 431-442. doi: 10.1016/j.sxmr.2020.01.001

Stanislavov, R., & Nikolova, V. (2003). Treatment of erectile dysfunction with pycnogenol and L-arginine. *J Sex Marital Ther, 29*(3), 207- 13. doi: 10.1080/00926230390155104

Stearns, V., Beebe, K., Iyengar, M., & Dube, E. (2003). Paroxetine controlled release in the treatment of menopausal hot flashes: A randomized controlled trial. *JAMA, 289*(21), 2827-34. doi: 10.1001/jama.289.21.2827

Stefanick, M., Anderson, G., Margolis, K., Hendrix, S., Rodabough, R., Paskett, E., … Chlebowski, R.; WHI Investigators. (2006). Effects of conjugated equine estrogens on breast cancer and mammography screening in postmenopausal women with hysterectomy. *JAMA, 295*(14), 1647-57. doi: 10.1001/jama.295.14.1647

Stein, D. (2008). Progesterone exerts neuroprotective effects after brain injury. *Brain Res Rev, 57*(2), 386-97.

doi: 10.1016/j.brainresrev.2007.06.012

Stein, D., Wright, D., & Kellermann, A. (2008). Does progesterone have neuroprotective properties? *Ann Emerg Med, 51*(2), 164-72. doi: 10.1016/j.annemergmed.2007.05.001

Steinauer, J., Waetjen, L., Vittinghoff, E., Subak, L., Hulley, S., Grady, D., ... Brown, J. (2005). Postmenopausal hormone therapy: Does it cause incontinence? *Obstet Gynecol, 106*(5 Pt 1), 940-5. doi: 10.1097/01.AOG.0000180394.08406.15

Stephenson, K., Price, C., Kurdowska, A., Neuenschwander, P., Stephenson, J., Pinson, B., ··· Bevan, M., (2004) Topical progesterone cream does not increase thrombotic and inflammatory factors in postmenopausal women. Blood, 104 (11), 5318.

Stoléru, S., Ennaji, A., Cournot, A., & Spira, A. (1993). LH pulsatile secretion and testosterone blood levels are influenced by sexual arousal in human males. *Psychoneuroendocrinology, 18*(3), 205-18. doi: 10.1016/0306-4530(93)90005-6

Stoll, B. (1999). Dietary supplements of dehydroepiandrosterone in relation to breast cancer risk. *Eur J Clin Nutr, 53*(10), 771-5. doi:

10.1038/sj.ejcn.1600889

Strain, G., Zumoff, B., Rosner, W., & Pi-Sunyer, X. (1994). The relationship between serum levels of insulin and sex hormone-binding globulin in men: The effect of weight loss. *J Clin Endocrinol Metab, 79*(4), 1173-6. doi: 10.1210/jcem.79.4.7962291

Su, C., & Lardy, H. (1991). Induction of hepatic mitochondrial glycerophosphate dehydrogenase in rats by dehydroepiandrosterone. *J Biochem, 110*(2), 207-13. doi: 10.1093/oxfordjournals.jbchem.a123558

Suh-Burgmann, E., Sivret, J., Duska, L., Del Carmen, M., & Seiden, M. (2003). Long-term administration of intravaginal dehydroepiandrosterone on regression of low-grade cervical dysplasia--a pilot study. *Gynecol Obstet Invest, 55*(1), 25-31. doi: 10.1159/000068953

Suvanto-Luukkonen, E., Koivunen, R., Sundström, H., Bloigu, R., Karjalainen, E., Häivä-Mällinen, L., & Tapanainen, J. (2005). Citalopram and fluoxetine in the treatment of postmenopausal symptoms: A prospective, randomized, 9-month, placebo-controlled, double-blind study. *Menopause, 12*(1), 18-26. doi: 10.1097/00042192-200512010-00006

The Coronary Drug Project. (1973). Findings leading to discontinuation of the 2.5-mg day estrogen group. The Coronary Drug Project Research Group. *JAMA, 226*(6),

652-7.

The Writing Group for the PEPI Trial. (1995). Effects of estrogen or estrogen/progestin regimens on heart disease risk factors in postmenopausal women. The Postmenopausal Estrogen/Progestin Interventions (PEPI) Trial. *JAMA, 273*(3), 199-208.

The Writing Group for the PEPI Trial. (1996). Effects of hormone therapy on bone mineral density: results from the postmenopausal estrogen/progestin interventions (PEPI) trial. *JAMA, 276*(17), 1389-96

Thijs, L., Fagard, R., Forette, F., Nawrot, T., & Staessen, J. (2003). Are low dehydroepiandrosterone sulphate levels predictive for cardiovascular diseases? A review of prospective and retrospective studies. *Acta Cardiol, 58*(5), 403-10. doi: 10.2143/AC.58.5.2005304

Thomas, T., Rhodin, J., Clark, L., & Garces, A. (2003). Progestins initiate adverse events of menopausal estrogen therapy. Climacteric. 2003 Dec;6(4):293-301

Titus-Ernstoff, L., Hatch, E., Hoover, R., Palmer, J., Greenberg, E., Ricker, W., ... Hartge P. (2001). Long-term cancer risk in women given diethylstilbestrol (DES) during pregnancy. *Br J Cancer, 84*(1), 126-33. doi: 10.1054/bjoc.2000.1521

Titus-Ernstoff, L., Troisi, R., Hatch, E., Wise, L.,

Palmer, J., Hyer, M., ... Hoover, R. (2006). Menstrual and reproductive characteristics of women whose mothers were exposed in utero to diethylstilbestrol (DES). *Int J Epidemiol,35*(4),862-8. doi: 10.1093/ije/dyl106

Tivesten, A., Hulthe, J., Wallenfeldt, K., Wikstrand, J., Ohlsson, C., & Fagerberg, B. (2006). Circulating estradiol is an independent predictor of progression of carotid artery intima-media thickness in middle-aged men. *J Clin Endocrinol Metab. 91*(11), 4433-7. doi: 10.1210/jc.2006-0932

Tivesten, A., Mellström, D., Jutberger, H., Fagerberg. B., Lernfelt, B., Orwoll, E., ... Ohlsson, C. (2007). Low serum testosterone and high serum estradiol associate with lower extremity peripheral arterial disease in elderly men. The MrOS Study in Sweden. *J Am Coll Cardiol, 50*(11), 1070-6. doi: 10.1016/j.jacc.2007.04.088

Tomaszewski, M., Charchar, F., Maric, C., Kuzniewicz, R., Gola, M., Grzeszczak, W., ... Zukowska-Szczechowska, E. (2009). Association between lipid profile and circulating concentrations of estrogens in young men. *Atherosclerosis, 203*(1), 257-62. doi: 10.1016/j.atherosclerosis.2008.06.002

Travison, T., Morley, J., Araujo, A., O'Donnell, A., &

McKinlay, J. (2006). The relationship between libido and testosterone levels in aging men. *J Clin Endocrinol Metab, 91*(7), 2509-13. doi: 10.1210/jc.2005-2508

Trunnel, J., Duffy, B., Marshall, V., Whitmore, W., & Woodard, H. (1951). The use of progesterone in treatment of cancer of the prostate. *J Clin Endocrinol Metab, 11*(7), 663-76. doi: 10.1210/jcem-11-7-663

Trunnel, J., Duffy, B., Marshall, V., Whitmore, W., & Woodard, H. (1950). The use of progesterone in treatment of cancer of the prostate. *J Clin Endocrinol Metab, 10*(7), 808.

Tsigos, C., & Chrousos, G. (2002). Hypothalamic-pituitary-adrenal axis, neuroendocrine factors and stress. *J Psychosom Res, 53*(4), 865-71. doi: 10.1016/s0022-3999(02)00429-4

Tulandi, T., Murphy, B., & Lal, S. (1985). Plasma cortisol concentrations in women with menopausal flushes. *Maturitas, 7*(4), 367-72. doi: 10.1016/0378-5122(85)90060-x

Tworoger, S., Missmer, S., Eliassen, A., Spiegelman, D., Folkerd, E., Dowsett, M., … Hankinson, S. (2006). The association of plasma DHEA and DHEA sulfate with breast cancer risk in predominantly premenopausal women. *Cancer Epidemiol Biomarkers Prev, 15*(5), 967-71. doi: 10.1158/1055-9965.EPI-05-0976

Tymchuk, C., Tessler, S., Aronson, W., & Barnard, R. (1998). Effects of diet and exercise on insulin, sex hormone-binding globulin, and prostate-specific antigen. *Nutr Cancer, 31*(2), 127-31. doi: 10.1080/01635589809514691

Urhausen, A., Albers, T., & Kindermann, W. (2004). Are the cardiac effects of anabolic steroid abuse in strength athletes reversible? *Heart, 90*(5), 496-501. doi: 10.1136/hrt.2003.015719

Vallée, M., Mayo, W., Darnaudéry, M., Corpéchot, C., Young, J., Koehl, M., ... Simon, H. (1997). Neurosteroids: deficient cognitive performance in aged rats depends on low pregnenolone sulfate levels in the hippocampus. *Proc Natl Acad Sci U S A, 94*(26), 14865-70. doi: 10.1073/pnas.94.26.14865

van Anders, S., Hamilton, L., Schmidt, N., & Watson, N. (2007). Associations between testosterone secretion and sexual activity in women. *Horm Behav, 51*(4), 477-82. doi: 10.1016/j.yhbeh.2007.01.003

Vashisht, A., Wadsworth, F., Carey, A., Carey, B., & Studd, J. (2005). A study to look at hormonal absorption of progesterone cream used in conjunction with transdermal estrogen. *Gynecol Endocrinol, 21*(2), 101-5. doi: 10.1080/09513590500128583

Verhoog, N., Allie-Reid, F., Vanden Berghe, W., Smith, C., Haegeman, G., Hapgood, J., & Louw, A. (2014). Inhibition of corticosteroid-binding globulin gene expression by glucocorticoids involves C/EBPβ. *PLoS One, 9*(10), e110702. doi: 10.1371/journal.pone.0110702

Vermeulen, A., Goemaere, S., & Kaufman, J. (1999). Testosterone, body composition and aging. *J Endocrinol Invest, 22*(5 Suppl), 110-6.

Villareal, D., & Holloszy, J. (2004). Effect of DHEA on abdominal fat and insulin action in elderly women and men: a randomized controlled trial. *JAMA, 292*(18), 2243-8. doi: 10.1001/jama.292.18.2243

Villareal, D., Holloszy, J., & Kohrt, W. (2000). Effects of DHEA replacement on bone mineral density and body composition in elderly women and men. *Clin Endocrinol (Oxf), 53*(5), 561-8. doi: 10.1046/j.1365-2265.2000.01131.x

Vitalone, A., Guizzetti, M., Costa, L., & Tita, B. (2003). Extracts of various species of Epilobium inhibit proliferation of human prostate cells. *J Pharm Pharmacol, 55*(5), 683-90. doi: 10.1211/002235703765344603

Vitalone, A., McColl, J., Thome, D., Costa, L., & Tita, B. (2003). Characterization of the effect of Epilobium extracts on human cell proliferation. *Pharmacology,* *69*(2), 79-87. doi: 10.1159/000072360

von Mühlen, D., Laughlin, G., Kritz-Silverstein, D., Bergstrom, J., & Bettencourt, R. (2008). Effect of dehydroepiandrosterone supplementation on bone mineral density, bone markers, and body composition in older adults: The DAWN trial. *Osteoporos Int, 19*(5), 699-707. doi: 10.1007/s00198-007-0520-z

Wald, M., Meacham, R., Ross, L., & Niederberger, C. (2006). Testosterone replacement therapy for older men. *J Androl, 27*(2), 126-32. doi: 10.2164/jandrol.05036

Walle, T., Otake, Y., Brubaker, J., Walle, U. & Halushka, P. (2001). Disposition and metabolism of the flavonoid chrysin in normal volunteers. *Br J Clin Pharmacol, 51*(2), 143-6. doi: 10.1111/j.1365-2125.2001.01317.x

Wan, M., Hunziker, P., & Kägi, J. (1993). Induction of metallothionein synthesis by cadmium and zinc in cultured rabbit kidney cells (RK-13). *Biochem J, 292*(Pt 2), 609-15. doi: 10.1042/bj2920609

Wang, C., Alexander, G., Berman, N., Salehian, B., Davidson, T., McDonald, V., … Swerdloff R. (1996). Testosterone replacement therapy improves mood in hypogonadal men--a clinical research center study. *J*
555

Clin Endocrinol Metab, 81(10), 3578-83. doi: 10.1210/jcem.81.10.8855804

Wang, P., Liao, S., Liu, R., Liu, C., Chao, H., Lu, SR., ... Liu, H. (2000). Effects of estrogen on cognition, mood, and cerebral blood flow in AD: a controlled study. *Neurology, 54*(11), 2061-6. doi: 10.1212/wnl.54.11.2061

Wang, S., Zhang, J., & Qie, L. (2014). Acupuncture relieves the excessive excitation of hypothalamic-pituitary-adrenal cortex axis function and correlates with the regulatory mechanism of GR, CRH, and ACTHR. *Evid Based Complement Alternat Med, 2014*, 495379. doi: 10.1155/2014/495379

Wang, S., Zhang, J., Yang, H., Wang, F., & Li, S. (2015). Acupoint specificity on acupuncture regulation of hypothalamic- pituitary-adrenal cortex axis function. *BMC Complement Altern Med, 15*, 87. doi: 10.1186/s12906-015-0625-4

Watts, N., Notelovitz, M., Timmons. M., Addison, W., Wiita, B., & Downey, L. (1995). Comparison of oral estrogens and estrogens plus androgen on bone mineral density, menopausal symptoms, and lipid-lipoprotein profiles in surgical menopause. *Obstet Gynecol, 85*(4), 529-37. doi: 10.1016/0029-7844(94)00448-m

Waynberg, J., & Brewer, S. (2000). Effects of herbal

vX on libido and sexual activity in premenopausal and postmenopausal women. *Adv Ther, 17*(5), 255-62. doi: 10.1007/BF02853164

Wehr, E., Pilz, S., Boehm, B., März, W., & Obermayer-Pietsch, B. (2010). Association of vitamin D status with serum androgen levels in men. *Clin Endocrinol (Oxf), 73*(2), 243-8. doi: 10.1111/j.1365-2265.2009.03777.x

Wei, Y., Dong, M., Zhong, L., Liu, J., Luo, Q., Lv, Y., … Dong, J. (2017). Regulation of hypothalamic-pituitary-adrenal axis activity and immunologic function contributed to the anti-inflammatory effect of acupuncture in the OVA-induced murine asthma model. *Neurosci Lett, 636*, 177-183. doi: 10.1016/j.neulet.2016.11.001

Weill-Engerer, S., David, J., Sazdovitch, V., Liere, P., Eychenne, B., Pianos, A., … Akwa, Y. (2002). Neurosteroid quantification in human brain regions: Comparison between Alzheimer's and nondemented patients. *J Clin Endocrinol Metab, 87*(11), 5138-43. doi: 10.1210/jc.2002-020878

Weisser, H., Tunn, S., Behnke, B., & Krieg, M. (1996). Effects of the sabal serrulata extract IDS 89 and its subfractions on 5 alpha-reductase activity in human benign prostatic hyperplasia. *Prostate, 28*(5), 300-6. doi: 10.1002/(SICI)1097-0045(199605)28:5<300:AID-

PROS5>3.0.CO;2-F

Welter, B., Hansen, E., Saner, K., Wei, Y., & Price, T. (2003). Membrane-bound progesterone receptor expression in human aortic endothelial cells. *J Histochem Cytochem, 51*(8), 1049-55. doi: 10.1177/002215540305100808

Westaby, D., Ogle, S., Paradinas, F., Randell, J., & Murray-Lyon, I. (1977). Liver damage from long-term methyltestosterone. *Lancet, 2*(8032), 262-3.

Whitcomb, B., Whiteman, M., Langenberg, P., Flaws, J., & Romani, W. (2007). Physical activity and risk of hot flashes among women in midlife. *J Womens Health (Larchmt), 16*(1), 124-33. doi: 10.1089/jwh.2006.0046

Whiteman, M., Staropoli, C., Langenberg, P., McCarter, R., Kjerulff, K., & Flaws, J. (2003). Smoking, body mass, and hot flashes in midlife women. *Obstet Gynecol, 101*(2), 264-72. doi: 10.1016/s0029-7844(02)02593-0

Whiting, P., Clouston, A., & Kerlin, P. (2002). Black cohosh and other herbal remedies associated with acute hepatitis. *Med J Aust, 177*(8), 440-3. doi: 10.5694/j.1326-5377.2002.tb04886.x

Wild, B., Brenner, J., Joos, S., Samstag. Y., Buckert, M., & Valentini, J. (2020). Acupuncture in persons with an increased stress level-Results from a random-ized-controlled pilot trial. *PLoS One, 15*(7), e0236004. doi: 10.1371/journal.pone.0236004

Williams, G., & Darbre, P. (2019). Low-dose environmental endocrine disruptors, increase aromatase activity, estradiol biosynthesis and cell proliferation in human breast cells. *Mol Cell Endocrinol, 486*, 55-64. doi: 10.1016/j.mce.2019.02.016

Woods, N., Carr, M., Tao, E., Taylor, H., & Mitchell, E. (2006). Increased urinary cortisol levels during the menopausal transition. *Menopause, 13*(2), 212-21. doi: 10.1097/01.gme.0000198490.57242.2e

Woods, N., Mitchell, E., & Smith-Dijulio, K. (2009). Cortisol levels during the menopausal transition and early postmenopause: Observations from the Seattle Midlife Women's Health Study. *Menopause, 16*(4), 708-18. doi: 10.1097/gme.0b013e318198d6b2

Wranicz, J., Cygankiewicz, I., Rosiak, M., Kula, P., Kula, K., & Zareba, W. (2005). The relationship between sex hormones and lipid profile in men with coronary artery disease. *Int J Cardiol, 101*(1), 105-10. doi: 10.1016/j.ijcard.2004.07.010

Wren, B. (2005). Transdermal progesterone creams for postmenopausal women: More hype than hope? *Med J Aust, 182*(5), 237-9. doi: 10.5694/j.1326-

5377.2005.tb06676.x

Wynder, J., Nicholson, T., DeFranco, D., & Ricke, W. (2015). Estrogens and male lower urinary tract dysfunction. *Curr Urol Rep, 16*(9), 61. doi: 10.1007/s11934-015-0534-6

Wysoczanski, M., Rachko, M., & Bergmann, S. (2008). Acute myocardial infarction in a young man using anabolic steroids. *Angiology, 59*(3), 376-8. doi: 10.1177/0003319707304883

Yan, M., Song, Y., Wong, C., Hardin, K., & Ho, E. (2008). Zinc deficiency alters DNA damage response genes in normal human prostate epithelial cells. *J Nutr, 138*(4), 667-73. doi: 10.1093/jn/138.4.667

Yassin, A., & Saad, F. (2007). Improvement of sexual function in men with late-onset hypogonadism treated with testosterone only. *J Sex Med, 4*(2), 497-501. doi: 10.1111/j.1743-6109.2007.00442.x

Yokota, M., Makita, K., Hirasawa, A., Iwata, T., & Aoki, D. (2016). Symptoms and effects of physical factors in Japanese middle-aged women. *Menopause, 23*(9), 974-83. doi: 10.1097/GME.0000000000000660

Yoon, B., Chin, J., Kim, J., Shin, M., Ahn, S., Lee, D., ... Na, D. (2018). Menopausal hormone therapy and mild cognitive impairment: A randomized, placebo-controlled trial. Menopause. 2018 Aug;25(8):870-876. doi: 10.1097/GME.0000000000001140

Yoshida, S., Honda, A., Matsuzaki, Y., Fukushima, S., Tanaka, N., Takagiwa, A., ... Salen, G. (2003). Anti-proliferative action of endogenous dehydroepiandrosterone metabolites on human cancer cell lines. *Steroids, 68*(1), 73-83. doi: 10.1016/s0039-128x(02)00117-4

Zaborowska, E., Brynhildsen, J., Damberg, S., Fredriksson, M., Lindh-Astrand, L., Nedstrand, E., ... Hammar, M. (2007). Effects of acupuncture, applied relaxation, estrogens and placebo on hot flushes in postmenopausal women: An analysis of two prospective, parallel, randomized studies. *Climacteric, 10*(1), 38-45. doi: 10.1080/13697130601165059

Zeleniuch-Jacquotte, A., Bruning, P., Bonfrer, J., Koenig, K., Shore, R., Kim, M., ... Toniolo, P. (1997). Relation of serum levels of testosterone and dehydroepiandrosterone sulfate to risk of breast cancer in postmenopausal women. *Am J Epidemiol, 145*(11), 1030-8. doi: 10.1093/oxfordjournals.aje.a009059

Zmuda, J., Cauley, J., Kriska, A., Glynn, N., Gutai, J., & Kuller, L. (1997). Longitudinal relation between endogenous testosterone and cardiovascular disease risk factors in middle-aged men. A 13-year follow-up of former Multiple Risk Factor Intervention Trial participants. *Am J Epidemiol, 146*(8), 609-17. doi: 10.1093/oxfordjournals.aje.a009326

Zwain, I., & Yen, S. (1999). Dehydroepiandrosterone: biosynthesis and metabolism in the brain. *Endocrinology, 140*(2), 880-7. doi: 10.1210/endo.140.2.6528